EBURY

LIVE YOUR

Dr Amrinder Bajaj is a senior gynaecologist presently affiliated to Fortis Memorial Research Institute (FMRI), Gurgaon. Formerly she was the head of the department of obstetrics and gynaecology at MAX, Patparganj, and a unit head at MAX Super Speciality Hospital, Shalimar Bagh, Delhi. She is a gold medallist and has done her post-graduation from All India Institute of Medical Sciences (AIIMS). Besides high-risk pregnancy and minimally invasive surgery, she has a special interest in menopause, on which she has given numerous talks to the medical fraternity and the lay public alike.

    She is also an award-winning author. She has written a memoir based on her association with the noted Indian author and columnist Khushwant Singh, two wellness books, an autobiographical novel, a novel based on the 1984 anti-Sikh riots, a textbook for nurses, a book of poems and a joke book. She has two columns in the magazine *Woman's Era* and regularly writes editorials, blog posts, travelogues, short stories and poems for magazines and newspapers like the *Times of India*, *Tribune* and *Indian Express*.

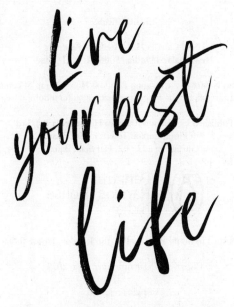

Live your best life

Understanding MENOPAUSE
for a Wiser, Happier and Healthier YOU

DR AMRINDER BAJAJ

EBURY
PRESS

An imprint of Penguin Random House

EBURY PRESS

USA | Canada | UK | Ireland | Australia
New Zealand | India | South Africa | China

Ebury Press is part of the Penguin Random House group of companies
whose addresses can be found at global.penguinrandomhouse.com

Published by Penguin Random House India Pvt. Ltd
4th Floor, Capital Tower 1, MG Road,
Gurugram 122 002, Haryana, India

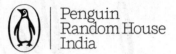

Penguin
Random House
India

First published in Ebury Press by Penguin Random House India 2022

ISBN 9780143451785

Typeset in Sabon LT Std by MAP Systems, Bengaluru, India
Printed at Thomson Press India Ltd, New Delhi

www.penguin.co.in

For
Sheetal Luthra,
literally,
my literary angel

Warning

When I am an old woman I shall wear purple,
With a red hat which doesn't go, and doesn't suit me.
And I shall spend my pension on brandy and summer gloves
And satin sandals, and say we've no money for butter.

I shall sit down on the pavement when I'm tired,
And gobble up samples in shops and press alarm bells,
And run my stick along the public railings
And make up for the sobriety of my youth . . .

—Jenny Joseph

'Way to go gal,' I would have told Jenny Joseph had I met her. Like her, I advise you to, 'Live your best life' after menopause *and* pay no heed to detractors for, 'A recent study discovered that women who carry a little extra weight live longer than the men who mention it.'

— Dr Amrinder Bajaj

Contents

INTRODUCTION

Female sex hormones are the blessing and the bane of a woman's life. A girl matures because the hormones deem it the right time to flood her system and are responsible for her burgeoning breasts and her curvy figure. A woman revels in her femineity, explores her sexuality, carries a baby in her womb, nurses an infant at her breast due to their presence in her body, in the right quantity at the right time. However, there are times when these hormones run amok, leading to menstrual irregularities, fibroids, polyps and even cancer. These issues need to be addressed by the custodians of the female reproductive tract—the gynaecologist. Finally, there comes a time in a woman's life when, the ovaries pack up and she attains what was dreaded all along—menopause. As soon as she enters her forties, she begins to have apprehensions about life without periods—periods that they gave her periodic problems—yet, she is reluctant to let go for periods are associated with youth. The clock cannot turn back and she has to learn how to live amicably in the present. I have written this book to clear misconceptions, to help the women tide over the difficult transition period and accept menopause gracefully. There is a fulfilling life after menopause; in fact, it is the best period of their lives, and one must learn to enjoy it.

A lot of women resent that their reproductive career is cut short by middle age, while men can reproduce till the end of their lives. 'Good riddance!' I say. Imagine having to worry about contraception and unwanted pregnancies at that age! After imposing upon the women the overwhelming responsibility of carrying forward the human race, Nature rewards them with a carefree existence after menopause. It is an exciting time, free from the responsibilities of child bearing/child-rearing and financial insecurities. Sexually, too, it can be a liberating period. Menopause is a gift that they ought to accept gratefully and utilize fully; especially now, with a longer life span, more and more women spend a third of their lives in the post-menopausal period.

Menopause brings with it some of the most significant changes in the women's life. It is the rite of passage into a new world where they can reclaim their life as an individual and, take up activities that give them pleasure, without feeling guilty. In most cases the transition from the reproductive to post-menopausal phase is smooth. Others have minor issues that can be addressed by lifestyle changes. For some, menopause can be a trying period with debilitating symptoms that require medical attention. However, it is important to note that *not all of us experience all the symptoms, all the time.*

The psychological impact of menopause is tremendous. There is a diminished sense of self-worth and jokes about her turning into a 'dried up prune' do not help. As it is, this 'Snow White' is trying hard to accommodate the seven dwarfs that have entered her life. Aptly named,

- Itchy
- Bitchy
- Sweaty
- Sleepy
- Bloated
- Forgetful
- Psycho

They become an unwanted part of her existence.

With the children exploring professional avenues and their own sexuality, usually away from home, time hangs heavy on her hands. As for her lesser halves (remember, the women are the better halves!), unable to understand the psychological impact of this massive change, they resort to ridiculing them to cover their ignorance. A caring partner would have made a difference but, being at the peak of their careers (some with a young mistress tucked on the side to reiterate *their* manhood), most men do not have time for an aging wife. She begins to think that menopause has made her less attractive to him. Why don't women realize that, with their receding hairline and preceding paunches, their male counterparts are no longer 'Prince Charming' they married? If *she* began to retaliate and joke about middle aged men who 'cannot get it up or keep it up', they would not stand a chance. All they want from them is a patient hearing, a kind word, a tender touch—actions that reassure us that despite these unasked-for changes in their bodies, they love and cherish them. It would cost them nothing but go a long way in restoring their sense of self-worth.

Instead of wallowing in self-pity in the pond of despondency, they should emerge from it gloriously like a lotus. A like-minded circle of friends, a hobby that one is passionate about and spiritual leanings come handy at this time of life. If you have neglected them, caring for a family that has ditched you now, this is the time to reconnect and bring good cheer back into your lives.

As a gynaecologist, who deals routinely with issues related to menopause, I was compelled to write this book to impress upon the reader's mind that, '**menopause is the end of menstruation, not the end of the world!**' I have given talks on this subject to both, the common public and the medical fraternity; and I was surprised to see that at the end of one such talk, a number of lady doctors—GPs, radiologists, physiotherapist, dentists (naturally no gynaecologists), flocked around me to seek remedies for issues like vaginal dryness leading to painful intercourse or passing urine on sneezing! If *this* was the level of ignorance amongst medical doctors, I can only begin to imagine the vast number of women out there who suffer in silence because they were too embarrassed to seek attention or think that these problems are a natural part of aging and accept them with resignation. This rekindled my desire to write this book for most of the issues related to menopause are amenable to treatment. An increase in our lifespan does not mean that, we should tolerate a decrease in the quality of our lives.

I have addressed these issues through the lives of three friends—Mona, a smart corporate head; Shiela, a portly school principal; and Meera, a happy-go-lucky homemaker. This is because they are real women facing real problems that any of us can relate to. No points for guessing on who I have fashioned the compassionate Dr Rosy on, to whom these three go for counselling and treatment!

Through this book, I will endeavour convert the formidable 'Menopause' into the delightful 'Me-No-Pause' so that you, my dear readers, achieve that level of joyful acceptance.

MENOPAUSE and ME NO PAUSE

'I'll shrivel you into a prune,' said Menopause.
'I will counter your assaults,' said Me No Pause.
'I'll break your bones.' said, Menopause.
'We'll see about that.' said, Me No Pause.
'I'll addle your brain and weaken your heart.'
'But can you weaken my spirit, you upstart?'
'I'll ravage you skin and thin your hair'
'Do you think that, for such trivia, I care?'
'I'll make you sad and cry without reason.'
'Don't you dare, try to commit such treason!'
'After hot flashes with cold sweats you'll shiver.'
'Is that the last arrow in your quiver?'
'A hundred ills within you, I'll let loose.'
'Yet, I know, this battle you will lose.'

C'mon now,
Stop playing the fiend and be my friend
And this stupid quarrel let us both end.
Menopause, show us your Jekyll side,
An endeavour to hide your horrible Hyde
Infighting please, I say, no more
Let's team up, and together win this war.

I am a part of you, and you are my part
Together, let's make a healthy start.
For now, Menopause and Me No Pause
Will fight together for a common cause
We have miles to go and years to live
And back to society, we've a lot to give.
With a husband married to his work
His decreasing demands, no longer irk
With children gone and elders gone
For myself alone, I am reborn
With sacrifice and drudgery, I'm done
Now, is the time to have some fun
So, behave yourself dear Menopause
And I promise,
Life will be a party, with no pause.'

                                        Dr Amrinder Bajaj

1

TURBULENCE

Perimenopause

Mona sat on a chair by the window, trying to read a book, but she couldn't concentrate. After a while, she gave up, snapped the book shut and stared into space with unseeing eyes. Her mind was elsewhere. She thought about her life in the years gone by and wondered if it was too late to change things around.

Mona was a self-assured corporate executive nearing her fortieth birthday. She had climbed the ladder of success solely by dint of her hard work and her decision-making acumen, and was proud of her career graph. However, the one casualty of her ambition had been her motherhood. She had deferred having children till she reached a point in her career when she felt secure about her position, but by the time she finally decided to start a family, her ovaries had refused to cooperate and a donor egg was not an option she cared for. 'If only I had had her eggs frozen well in time, maybe . . .' she thought for a moment. But deciding to focus on the positives, at least for that day, she moved on from that thought. Whom was she kidding? With the thankless, unending responsibility of bringing up children, she could not have given her best to the profession that had given her so much satisfaction, she told herself firmly.

Mona had always been an overachiever, surpassing targets, earning accolades and bonuses, but in the recent past, she had begun to observe some changes within herself. She could feel her body and her mind slowing down. There was nothing to worry about yet, she knew, but the niggling disquiet that had begun to shadow her could not be wished away. She still took major corporate decisions and carried out all her initiatives as a department head with great enthusiasm. However, of late, the threat of impending menopause had begun to haunt her. From what she knew, she would lose her looks and the admiring glances men gave her would soon be directed towards others. Her skin would wrinkle, her hair would grey and her breasts would sag. What then? Skin tightening creams and frequent visits to the beauty parlour and the hair colouring salon would provide, at best, camouflage. There was no reversing the ageing process.

She had even begun to forget names. If her memory loss progressed, she would stand nowhere. The corporate world was a cruel world, and they would replace her in a jiffy—she had seen it happen with others. Their modus operandi were to make things so difficult for the person they wanted to get rid of that they would be forced to resign. People who were not driven enough to burn the candle at both ends in this cut-throat world were eased out in this manner, but she could never imagine such a thing happening to her. In her desperation, she downloaded an app called 'What to Expect when Expecting Menopause'. She would apprehensively await the symptoms described and thought that she could actually circumvent vaginal dryness by keeping herself hydrated!

Once again, she tried to enter the world inhabited by the characters in the book but could not take her mind off the mess she had made of her own life. In a desperate attempt to hang on to her youth, she had a torrid affair with her immediate subordinate, Dhruv. She needed the reassurance of male attention, of being told how wonderful and smart she was, and Dhruv knew exactly how to please her. Though she did not love him, and she knew that he did it all for professional gain and it could all backfire horribly on her, she could not help herself. In her heart, she knew that she loved her kind and caring husband, Mohit. He had never blamed her for her inability to conceive even though he adored children, and that made her hate herself even more. Forbidden sex had become an addiction that she could not resist, but guilt would leach away whatever pleasure she got from it.

After a couple of months of hollow joy, what she had dreaded all along came to pass. Dhruv started becoming overbearing and demanding. He asked for an out-of-turn promotion and issued veiled threats about making their affair public if she did not comply. There was no way she could extricate herself from this web of deceit and blackmail. Plus, the hot flashes caused by perimenopausal hormonal changes that had begun to plague her now made her angry, and the cold sweats that followed were partly due to the fear of being exposed. Dhruv had become a Frankensteinian monster of her own making, who was out to destroy all that she held sacred and dear. Things seemed to be falling apart and she did not know how to control them.

Reduced to a bundle of nerves, she could not sleep for nights on end. She had lost her appetite and her peace of mind, and people began to comment on her tired and drawn looks. There were dark circles under her eyes and her clothes hung loose on her. She dared not contemplate the consequences of her actions. She imagined herself sitting disgraced and discarded amid the shards of her shattered life. There would be no option left but the cowardly act of suicide if the current situation persisted. She was grateful for the fact that she would not leave orphaned children behind. The image of her devastated husband, who did not deserve the humiliation she would bring upon him, would be the cross she would carry to the grave with her.

One night, the dam broke. She sat huddled on her bed, her head on her knees, which were drawn to her chest. Huge sobs wracked her form as tears coursed steadily down her cheeks. Mohit got up with a start. Mona was not one to cry easily, so he was taken aback. She usually vented by raving and ranting. This display of sorrow alarmed him. He reached out, put his arms around her and drew her to his heart; he rocked her gently back and forth till her tears subsided.

'Oh god, what have I done?' she thought. Heaven was being in his arms and she had spurned to satisfy a whim. If only she could turn back time and erase that chapter from her life . . .

'Is there anything you want to tell me?' Mohit asked gently, pouring out a glass of water. She sat back on the pillow and gulped it. He stood still, looking at her. More tears rolled down her cheeks, but she wiped them away fiercely. She *had* to confront this, the consequences be damned! Divorce or death. She could no longer continue in a state of torment and told Mohit all that had transpired. There was a stunned silence. Mohit sat down with a thump in front of her and, with a stricken look on his face, a look that Mona would not forget till her dying day, asked, 'Where have I gone wrong?'

'It's not about you at all!' she gave an anguished cry. 'You are the best husband a woman could wish for. *I* have destroyed the sanctity of our marriage.'

'But why?'

'I don't know, Mohit . . . maybe I was trying to hold on to my youth. I had begun to experience changes in my body that I was unable to accept. I felt unattractive . . . still do . . .' she broke off. She knew that this was barely any reason for her to have done what she did and yet, that was how she'd felt.

'And you do not love that, that . . .'

'I hate him with all my heart. I could kill him with my bare hands. I love you, and look what I have done to you! I was contemplating suicide . . . I have hurt you badly and I do not know how to make amends . . .'

They went to a marriage counsellor, who told them it was all about midlife crisis and the insecurities that come with it. Thankfully, Mohit understood. He was still in love with his wife and wanted to preserve their marriage. So, together, they began the business of repairing things: Dhruv was put in his place when Mohit confronted him and had himself transferred to another unit as fast as he could.

Next on their agenda was a visit to the gynaecologist to discuss the physical changes that Mona had been experiencing, but was dismissing them as stress related. Once they were in the doctor's chamber, Mona talked about her fear of approaching menopause. Dr Rosy Dua listened carefully. When Mona finished, the first thing the doctor made her do was delete that app from her phone right there and then. She laughed at the novel way Mona had found of preventing vaginal dryness!

'I wish it were as easy to deal with as this app suggests. It's not about drinking more water—the excess water will just be flushed out by the kidneys. Moreover, it is not about hydration at all! With the depletion of hormones, the vagina thins out, losing its elasticity and moistness. If and when the situation arises (mind you, not all women experience all the symptoms of menopause), I will prescribe oestrogen cream to make your vagina as supple as before.'

'You will?' asked Mona, smiling with relief.

'I can prescribe something even better!'

'What is it?' asked Mona eagerly.

'The most enjoyable way to keep your vagina lubricated is to have regular sex for as many years as you can.'

'That I will,' said Mona with delight. 'But tell me, doctor, I am still menstruating. Why have I started having symptoms of menopause, like mood swings? I have even begun to forget names, for instance.'

'You are going through what we call perimenopause. You see, menopause is preceded by varying periods of perimenopause before the periods stop altogether. During this time, periods become irregular, heavier or lighter than usual, infrequent with erratic gaps or stop altogether at once. Many menopausal symptoms begin in the perimenopausal period, causing confusion and concern.

'One thing I want you to remember is that irregular periods, especially heavy flow with clots, frequent periods and inter-menstrual bleeding (bleeding between periods), especially after intercourse, may **not** be due to perimenopause. In that case, we would have to look for a cause, which could be anything from fibroids to polyps or endometrial hyperplasia (thickened inner lining of the uterus, which could be precancerous) and cancers. So please do not think that every sort of abnormal uterine bleeding is due to menopause and let it pass. A visit to the gynaecologist is necessary to rule out any other problems.'

'I'll keep that in mind,' Mona said, getting the seriousness of the issue. She had been taking things lightly.

'Another thing I want to warn you about,' said the doctor, 'is that many times, women get careless about contraception and think that the delay in periods is due to menopausal changes, when to their horror, they learn that they are pregnant! One must continue using contraception for at least two years after the periods have stopped to prevent such an occurrence.'

'Contraception plays no role in my life whatsoever,' stated Mona categorically. 'Initially, we had delayed childbearing till it was too late. The infertility expert told us that the quality of my eggs had deteriorated with age, and I could get pregnant only with donor eggs. Though he is very fond of kids, my husband wanted *our* child and not his child with some unknown woman's gene pool, so we gave up the idea.'

'You never know,' smiled Dr Rosy, not realizing that her words would prove prophetic one day, but Mona appeared preoccupied. Her memory lapses had begun to play on her mind.

'What is it?' asked the doctor.

'As I told you earlier, I have begun to forget names. Is that a sign of Alzheimer's?' asked Mona fearfully.

'If you remember that you do not remember, you don't have Alzheimer's.'

'Thank God!' Mona heaved a sigh of relief.

'We all begin to forget things as we age,' continued the doctor. 'The other day, as we sat at the dining table, I told my son, "*Wahan se woh pakda do* (Give me that from there)." Though he knew full well what I wanted and from where, he asked, "*Kahan se kya pakda do* (What from where)?" and laughed when I struggled to remember the name,' said Dr Rosy.

Mona broke into peals of laughter. She had not imagined that she would enjoy a medical consult so much.

Dr Rosy conducted a thorough general physical examination and an internal check-up, which revealed no abnormality. After this, she advised a battery of tests and asked Mona to come back with the reports: a Pap smear, an ultrasound and a mammography; blood tests to check her levels of haemoglobin, thyroid and sugar, a lipid profile, a liver and a kidney function test, and X-ray and ECG.

'Why, you are as fit as a twenty-year-old!' said the doctor when Mona returned with the reports for a follow-up consult, which pleased Mona no end. 'But you *must* come for yearly preventive health check-ups so that diseases can be diagnosed and treated at the earliest.'

'Yes, ma'am!'

'Also, examine your breasts for lumps every month after your periods as I have taught you, and teach it to all the women you know. You will be doing them a great service, for breast cancer is the number one killer among females these days. If caught early, it is curable.'

'I definitely will, doctor.'

'I am prescribing calcium tablets which you must take daily as bones lose calcium with age, which makes them brittle and prone to fractures. You must have heard of frail old ladies breaking their bones after a mere fall in the bathroom. People as well-endowed as me . . .' said the doctor and smiled, though her weight was just a bit above normal, '. . . have fat to cushion our falls and therefore have a lower chance of fractures, though we are more prone to high blood pressure, diabetes and heart problems!' Mona laughed but the doctor was serious. 'The incidence of heart problems also increases after menopause. This is because female hormones protect a woman against heart disease as long as she is menstruating. Once the reproductive phase of her life is over, the levels of these hormones decrease, and a female is as much at risk for a heart attack as her male counterparts.'

'And Vitamin D deficiency?' asked Mona. 'We hear so much about it these days.'

'Vitamin D is necessary for the absorption of calcium. It is a shame that Vitamin D deficiency is rampant in a country flooded with sunshine. We sit in air-conditioned homes, offices, cars and malls, and avoid the sun like the plague or slather sunscreen on exposed areas when we do venture out.'

'True,' agreed Mona.

'I had once gone to Nice in France with my husband and on the pebbled beach lay bikini-(un)clad women, for most had taken off their bikini tops, soaking in the sun, wanting to acquire a tan that we desperately avoid; it seems no one is satisfied with what God gives us! The clear waters of the Mediterranean stretched out as far as the eye could see. I had never seen so many shades of blue in a single expanse of water and excitedly I said to my husband, "Isn't the scenery beautiful?"

'"It is indeed!" said my husband, ogling the near-naked women; he wasn't looking at the sea at all!'

Mona burst out laughing. The doctor did have a sense of humour and Mona found herself liking her more by the minute.

'We'll get your Vitamin D levels tested. I will prescribe it only if necessary, for hypervitaminosis of D is a dangerous thing, because the excess collects in the body while extra doses of other vitamins are excreted by the kidney.'

'Okay . . .' said Mona, realizing the harmful effects of self-medication.

'The important thing is not to let yourself stagnate mentally and physically. Though you look wonderfully fit and beautiful for your age, it is important to keep yourself busy with things that you enjoy, besides your work. Some sort of exercise and recreation is a must.'

'I have a high-powered job; I swim regularly and have very good friends,' said Mona, pleased with the compliment.

'Then you are on the right track. Don't take yourself too seriously and learn to enjoy life.'

'Sure, doctor!' said Mona, laughing happily.

'If this lady, with the tremendous stress of her profession, can laugh at her own menopausal symptoms and carry on with life cheerfully, why can't I?' thought Mona. 'If I could age half as gracefully as her and retain my zest for life, I will have nothing to fear.'

'Thank you, doctor, thank you very much!' gushed Mona, vigorously shaking her hand. 'You have saved my life!'

'Isn't this a bit melodramatic?' said Dr Rosy, arching an eyebrow.

'You don't know half the story, doctor. Maybe, someday, I will tell you when we get to know each other better.

Life has given me a second chance and I am not going to waste a minute of it.'

'*Ja Simran ja, jee le apni zindagi* (Go Simran go, live your life),' laughed the doctor, mouthing the famous dialogue from the movie *Dilwale Dulhania Le Jayenge*.

'I definitely will, and in a happier frame of mind,' laughed Mona.

'There are so many women out there in this transitional phase of life, struggling silently with their fears and phobias, but are too embarrassed to visit a doctor for "nothing in particular",' said the doctor thoughtfully. 'They do not know where to turn, whom to ask. Every symptom, big or small, is attributed to menopause, especially by older women in their lives, whose advice these troubled women usually seek, when a few months' delay can convert an operable cancer to something beyond cure. As for Google, the less said the better . . .'

'Yes,' said Mona, 'the first thing women like me do is google.'

'We are fed up competing with Dr Google,' said Dr Rosy. 'Some doctors have put up a notice in their clinics stating that those who come to them for a second consult after visiting Dr Google will be charged double. That is why I was thinking . . .'

Mona laughed and waited for her to go on.

'I was wondering if your colleagues or friends would be interested in a talk, or perhaps an informal discussion, on this issue by a professional . . .'

'That is an excellent idea! I will definitely discuss it with my colleagues,' said Mona happily. 'After just one meeting with you, I have realized that menopause is no longer the demon in the dark that I feared. Thanks to you, I go home vastly relieved.'

Her equilibrium restored, Mona began to anticipate and accept this phase of life instead of resenting and fighting it. Her love for her husband welled and overflowed. Mohit and the doctor had pulled the real Mona out from the tangle of nerves she had become to a happier and a calmer person. All was well with her world again and she could only raise her hands heavenwards in a thankful prayer.

Her 'walking' colony friends Meera and Shiela noticed the spring had returned to her step and the twinkle to her eyes. They were glad to have their old Mona back. The moody, irritable person they had walked with in the past few months was not the Mona they knew. Attempts to draw her out had failed and they had given up on her but now, the Mona who appeared from behind the clouds was as radiant as the full moon! Whatever troubled her had been dealt with effectively, it seemed, and they were both happy for her.

'Guess where Mohit is taking me next week,' said Mona, out of the blue.

'Where?' they asked in unison.

'Maldives, for a second honeymoon.'

'But weren't you supposed to go abroad later, on your wedding anniversary?' asked Shiela.

'Mohit surprised me by advancing it! Who am I to complain?'

'You are one lucky girl,' said Meera with a tinge of envy.

'That I am,' she replied.

If only they knew how lucky!

Friendly advice: Don't be afraid of menopause. The more you understand your symptoms and yourself, the easier it will be to control.

2

THE HOT FLASHES AND COLD SWEATS

A mixed group of about twenty-odd women, ranging in age from thirty-five to about fifty-eight, were gathered in the seminar room of Mascot Enterprises, and it was not for a presentation. Mona had taken her boss' permission to have Dr Rosy over to talk to all of them. She was going to advise and help no-nonsense women who, in their high-profile jobs, did not look like they needed any help! But Mona knew they were all going through things, just like her. They may have climbed the ladder of success in their departments but inside, they were as insecure as the woman on the street who needed help to tide over the 'midlife crisis'. Dr Rosy was just who they needed. She had deliberately asked for a smaller group so that the interaction would be intimate and had filtered people by age so that they could figure out solutions together.

The women in the room, however, did not know this. They looked at each other uncertainly, fake smiles plastered to their faces, some made flippant remarks to cover their nervousness, and others pretended nonchalance, saying they had come just to please Mona. All were worried though, wondering how much of their 'ageing issues' should they reveal. They knew that in the highly-westernized upper class Indian society, where the young and youth were worshipped, growing old was a crime and people would think less of you as you aged.

Dr Rosy Dua came into the room like breath of fresh air. In her pink sari, with a sprig of jasmine in her hair, she won them over with her radiant smile. Mona introduced her to her colleagues, after which all the ladies, thick or thin, tall or short, pretty or plain, in saris, skirts or business suits, introduced themselves one by one.

The introductions over, Dr Rosy began, 'Thanks to Mona, I am honoured to meet such a lovely group of ladies who personify the adage "beauty with brains".' Everyone relaxed and smiled. Maybe it wasn't going to be that bad after all!

'The same holds true for you too, doctor,' said Mona, smiling.

'Thank you,' said Dr Rosy and smiled. 'At the outset, I would like to tell you that all of us here are just women, women who have left their designations at their desks. I have brought mine along because it is my day, like it will be Sheetal's on the day there is a meeting on customer care, and Leena's when marketing issues are to be discussed. Do you agree?'

'Yes!' they chorused.

'And we will all use first names. Feel free to call me Rosy.'

They smiled and nodded.

'Just give me five minutes to introduce our new friend "menopause" before we proceed with an informal chat. We all know that menopause means the stopping of our periods, but this doesn't happen suddenly. It occurs in stages. Imagine that menopause is a temperamental creature, like most of us, but if handled right, she will serve us well. It is in our interests to treat her well for, whether we like it or not, she has come to stay with us for the rest of our lives. The nature of menopause differs in different women. With some, she becomes instant friends, with others, she takes time to get acquainted, and with a few, she remains at loggerheads till the gynaecologist steps in to set matters right. Temperamental or easy-going, one thing is for sure— slowly, insidiously, she tries to take over our systems one by one and if we are not vigilant, she will be running (ruining) over lives before we realize it. Don't let her get the better of you! Seek medical help sooner rather than later, before the situation gets out of hand. As a permanent guest whom we are reluctantly trying to assimilate into our lives, we are totally within our rights to put her in her place if she misbehaves. Got it?' asked Dr Rosy.

There was a chorus of 'Yes, ma'am!' from the group, which was gratifying.

'As we know, the only constant in life is change, more so for women. Female hormones at every milestone—be it puberty, pregnancy, abortion, delivery or breast feeding— cause upheavals that create havoc, but they finally settle down. During menopause, the depletion of hormones bring about a different set of changes, which may take some time to adjust to. No one should grudge you that adjustment period. As we have adjusted to strangers who become family after marriage, to motherhood, to the demise of our parents, with our infinite capacity for resilience, we will eventually adjust to menopause and learn to become comfortable in our own skins, even if they are dry, wrinkled and loose,' said Dr Rosy, who saw before her twenty sets of attentive ears, interested eyes and tentative smiles.

'The word "menopause" is derived from Greek—"menos" meaning "month" and "pausis" meaning "to stop". Now let me explain with the help of slides:

Definition

Menopause is the cessation of menstruation for a period of twelve months or more, in a healthy woman over forty-five years old who is not on the pill. It is a retrospective clinical diagnosis which, in other words means, that only after a woman has stopped menstruating for a year, will she know that she has attained menopause. It occurs when the ovaries stop producing the female sex hormones oestrogen and progesterone.

Classification

- Natural menopause: is a normal part of the ageing process, usually occurring between forty-four and fifty-two years of age
- Premature menopause: occurring before the age of forty
- Delayed menopause: occurring after the age of fifty-four
- Medical menopause: due to radiotherapy/chemotherapy in cancers

♦ Surgical menopause: when the ovaries have been removed surgically

Symptoms of menopause

Some women have no symptoms whatsoever. In fact, they enjoy the benefits of menopause, which include:

♦ No menstrual bleeding or cramps
♦ No PMS (premenstrual syndrome)
♦ No anaemia due to excessive bleeding
♦ No unwanted pregnancies
♦ No need for contraception (after two years from the cessation of periods)
♦ Increased libido (sex drive) in some

Symptomatic menopausal women could have one or more of the following:

♦ Hot flashes and cold sweats
♦ Vaginal dryness that can affect sex life
♦ Urinary complaints: frequency, burning, inability to hold urine, leakage on coughing and sneezing
♦ Mood swings, forgetfulness
♦ Weight gain despite eating the same amount of food
♦ Skin changes: itching, dryness, warts, wrinkles
♦ Hair thins out on the head but may appear on the chin and/or upper lip!
♦ Fatigue

Yearly preventive health check-ups are a must, even if you feel perfectly normal, for early detection and/or follow-up of health problems, for menopause predisposes women to

- ◆ Heart diseases
- ◆ Fractures
- ◆ Cancers

If these conditions are diagnosed before they have caused damage, the quality and "quantity" of life improves drastically.

Doubts, however negligible, symptoms, however trivial, must be discussed with the doctor. After a thorough general physical check-up, which includes blood pressure measurements, examination of your chest, abdomen, breasts and a pelvic examination, you will be sent to the other departments for heart, eye and dental examinations, which will be followed by tests such as:

- ◆ CBC for measuring your haemoglobin levels
- ◆ Blood sugars: fasting and after meals
- ◆ Thyroid, heart, kidney, liver function tests
- ◆ X-ray
- ◆ ECG
- ◆ Ultrasound
- ◆ Pap smear for early detection of cancer or precancerous changes in the cervix (mouth of the uterus)
- ◆ Mammography for breast lumps
- ◆ Bone densitometry for bone health

From the number of tests required, you must have gauged that almost every system in our body is affected by the depletion of female sex hormones and advancing age.

You will also be taught to self-examine your breasts, and any lump you feel should be reported to your doctor, even if painless—especially if painless. A foul-smelling vaginal discharge which may or may not be blood-tinged calls for a gynaecological consult. Irregular, heavy flow and inter-menstrual bleeding should also be looked into. *Bleeding after menopause or after intercourse is absolutely not acceptable* and must be tackled at once for it could be due to cancer! Women often shy away from discussing such an embarrassing complaint or take it in their stride thinking it is due to menopause. Those of you who are less than forty-five years of age can get yourselves vaccinated against cervical cancer. In fact, I recommend getting all the females in the family between the ages of nine and forty-five vaccinated.

Remember, **menopause is the end of menstruation, not the end of the world.** It is, in fact, a gateway to a whole new world that can be best enjoyed by adopting the following measures:

♦ A balanced, nutritious diet that includes soya foods, adequate calcium and vitamin D; avoid caffeine, smoking, alcohol and spicy foods, and keep your weight in check. The last is easier said than done but important, nevertheless.

♦ Exercise reduces hot flashes, improves sleep and boosts mood. Weight-bearing exercises keep bones strong while Kegel exercises strengthen vaginal muscles and prevent leakage of urine. Relaxation techniques such as yoga and meditation are important for peace of mind for one should strive for overall health—physical, mental, emotional and spiritual.

- ◆ Clothes: dress lightly and in layers, wear loose clothes at night and sleep on cotton sheets in a cool, well-ventilated room.
- ◆ Intimacy: remain sexually active for an increased sense of well-being.
- ◆ Medical: go for yearly preventive health check-ups, manage medical problems like blood pressure, diabetes and cholesterol and report untoward symptoms like postmenopausal or post-coital bleeding.

* * *

'This much talk is enough for today,' concluded Dr Rosy, switching off the slide show. 'Now let's get to the fun part. We'll take up a common symptom, the one most of us tend to experience at this time of our lives, and beat the daylights out of it. Agreed?'

'Yes!' they all said.

'Those who suffer from hot flashes and cold sweats raise your hands.'

Even as they looked at each other uncertainly, to their utter surprise, Dr Rosy raised her hand! Reluctantly, then with more confidence, one by one, eight women raised their hands.

'How does it feel, Mala?' asked Dr Rosy.

'I feel a sort of heat rising to my face from my neck, making me feel all hot and flustered. A little while later, I break into a sweat and start shivering.'

'You have summed up the symptoms beautifully. What do you do about it?'

'What can I do?'

'Anything anyone suggests to help you?' she asked.

'Yes. My husband tells me to sit in the fridge and his sister tells me to grin and bear it instead of cribbing all the time.'

'Hah! You should have punched the brother and the sister in the face,' said Dr Rosy indignantly. Everyone laughed and the atmosphere around them lightened. 'I know exactly how it feels,' she added.

When she said that, many of the others also started sharing.

'My husband too makes fun of me,' fumed Aparna. 'If it was "that time of her month" when I suffered from premenstrual syndrome, now it is "that time of her life". I feel like banging the saucepan on his head!'

'You should have. That was exactly what I was going to prescribe! The hot flash of anger and cold fury he will experience after such an attack will make him understand what you are going through. Women, especially of our age, cannot be taken lightly!'

They all laughed, and it felt like the ice had been broken within this group.

'Would anyone else like to share her experience?' asked Dr Rosy.

'My husband switches off the AC and I switch it on again. This goes on throughout the night and both of us get up grumpy and irritable in the morning. I tell him to use a blanket, but he insists on torturing me,' said Malvika. 'I would have shifted to the other room if it did not worsen our relationship.'

'I wish they would be more understanding,' murmured Dr Rosy sympathetically. 'As for me, I sweat so much in the operation theatre that the OT staff lowers the temperature of the AC for this "hot lady" whenever I have a case!'

'That you certainly are, doctor!' gushed Sheetal with mounting appreciation.

'I parody the song "*Mausam hai ashiqana*" and sing "*mausam hai menopausal*" when the weather becomes hot and then cold by turns at the change of the seasons,' continued Dr Rosy, much to their amusement.

'The internet is full of horrible cartoons about women with hot flashes, but it's best to ignore them,' she continued. 'Let's understand why they occur and how to manage them. The reduction of hormones in the premenopausal period (the period before menopause) and the absence of hormones after menopause affects the thermoregulatory system (body's temperature control system), besides almost all other systems. This leads to hot flashes and cold sweats.'

'So what do we do about them?' asked Mala, eager to learn about their management.

'They usually happen because of stress, worry or excitement. Avoid situations that make you feel too emotional (easier said than done!), vigorous exercises, spicy foods and going out in the heat. Other ways to manage this distressful condition are:

- ◆ Take a cold drink at the first sign of a flush
- ◆ Perform deep breathing exercises
- ◆ Meditate
- ◆ A cool shower at bedtime decreases night sweats
- ◆ Use cotton sheets and lingerie which absorb perspiration

And, do not sit in the fridge!'

While the others laughed, Pushpa, the lady in black at the back, appeared sad. Clearly, it was no laughing matter for her.

'What is it, Pushpa?' asked Dr Rosy gently.

Pushpa looked up. There were tears in her eyes.

'Pushpa, I hate tears!' Dr Rosy mouthed the famous Rajesh Khanna dialogue from *Amar Prem*. 'Tell me what is making you so upset. After all, I have come to help you.'

At this, her restraint broke and Pushpa collapsed in a torrent of tears. Ending the session quickly, Dr Rosy had the place emptied so that Pushpa could have the privacy she needed to confide in the doctor. The poor woman had about twenty-five to thirty episodes of hot flashes each day, which made her miserable and incapable of any productive work. This led to poor performance at work and a warning from her boss to pull up her socks or else . . . and she was at her wits' end. She thought it was something that came along with menopause and there was nothing she could do about it.

'But there is medical help for you!' exclaimed Dr Rosy. 'You meet me in the office. After I examine you and run some tests, I will put you on Hormone Replacement Therapy (HRT) for some time and you will be perfectly fine.'

'You really think so?' asked Pushpa, looking up at her through a film of tears.

'Though we have stopped using HRT for most other symptoms, they are still being used effectively in uncontrolled hot flashes. Just you wait and see.'

Friendly advice: Now is as good a time as ever to get into a healthy routine. Regular diet and exercise will help with most symptoms.

3

THAT EMBARRASSING LEAK
Stress Incontinence

Shiela, Mona and Meera were the best of friends. Shiela ran a nursery school, Mona was a corporate executive and Meera was a homemaker. Mona was the smartest of the three. She wore hip-hugging jeans with sneakers that looked great on her youthful figure, even though she was in her early forties. Maybe it was because she had never had children, thought the other two enviously.

Meera was happy-go-lucky. Her figure, though a bit on the plump side, was good enough, as was her complexion. She wore salwar-kameez with sports shoes and carried a small towel in her hand to wipe the sweat off her face.

Shiela, was fifty-two years of age and overweight, always wore sarees and glasses and walked with a slight limp due to arthritis in one knee. She was the principal of a nursery school and had great administrative skills, with which she managed her school, her home and her two daughters-in-law. Her widowed mother married her off at eighteen, as soon she got the first marriage proposal for her daughter. Though Shiela had two sons in quick succession soon after her marriage, her progressive husband made her complete her graduation and a nursery teacher training course. He opened a one room nursery school for her in their own premises which had flourished, and was now a prestigious primary school of which, Shiela was very proud. She had an intimidating, no-nonsense air about her, but revealed her soft and funny side to her friends.

Despite the differences in their temperaments and jobs, the three had become the best of friends. In the evenings, they forgot about their responsibilities and became who they truly were inside—fun-loving girls! They had made friends with each other while walking in the park and had become inseparable since then. Their routine consisted of an hour of brisk walking in the evening, followed by half-an-hour's relaxation on a park bench where they discussed their day. There was nothing much that they did not know about each other. They had matured together, raised their children and discussed the issues that bothered them. In the early years, they had vented against orthodox, rigid, demanding mothers-in-law. Now that the tables had turned, Shiela found *her* daughters-in-law lazy and disrespectful, when in fact *they* were terrified of her! Mona's mother-in-law had expired; Meera's had been reduced to a frailer, gentler version of herself and the two women had now grown to love each other as mother and daughter.

Meera had three daughters, the last one forced upon her by her mother-in-law, desperate for a grandson.

However, what had been a difficult phase for her with three children became a boon as the girls grew up. The girls doted on her, as did her sons-in-law. Her husband was a businessman and an introvert. When at home, he read the newspaper from cover-to-cover, watched the news on TV in English and revised it all over again in Hindi, oblivious of her presence. He took for granted the fact that his needs were anticipated and met. After feeling hurt in the initial years, Meera the chatterbox, had become used to it by now. In fact, she wouldn't know what to say to him if he suddenly became talkative. For her, her friends became the outlet. They gossiped, watched movies and went shopping together. She rarely missed her evening walk except when her daughters visited with her grandchildren. However, these days, she was absenting herself quite often and this had puzzled the other two. Each time they asked her the reason for her not joining them, Meera gave a vague answer, which was unlike her.

Unknown to them, it had all started when she had suddenly stopped menstruating at the age of forty-seven. She was glad when it happened because it meant the end of the many problems related with periods. Menopause had been kind to her and she wondered what the fuss was all about. Then one day, it happened. She was watching a comedy show on TV and laughed out loud at one of the stand-up comedian's straight-faced one-liners, only to realize, to her horror, that she had wet her panties. Over time, the situation became worse. She dreaded laughing or coughing or even sneezing. Every sneeze and bout of coughing brought about a leakage of urine. As if this was not enough, she could not control the urge to pass urine and barely managed to reach the toilet in time. She even felt that she smelled of urine, which made her very conscious of going out. What if Shiela cracked one of her hilarious jokes? She could not risk peeing in her panties right there in front of them. She looked it up online, only to come across a cruel bit of humour, 'Midlife is when I have to change my underwear after every sneeze', and shut it down in disgust.

At her wits' end, she went to their family doctor, who suggested that she get her blood sugars and urine tested. They were normal. What now? She was told to do Kegel's exercises regularly but contracting her vaginal muscles day in and day out did not help. Her incontinence was beyond the purview of mere exercises. As her symptoms increased, she began to withdraw from her social circle and became a recluse. No parties, no satsang, not even the evening walk with friends she so looked forward to. All she wanted was to be near a toilet in a maxi without underwear so that whenever she felt the need to urinate, she had but to take a few steps, lift her dress and sit on the pot. Peeing without wetting her clothes was an achievement and her life began to revolve around it. She would have been reduced to a nervous wreck had it not been for Shiela and Mona. They had not seen her for a week, so one evening, they came barging in. Meera was very happy to see them.

'Why don't you come for a walk these days?' asked Shiela.

'I have not been keeping well,' she lied.

'What happened?'

'Nothing serious; just a headache, body ache and fever.' She was too embarrassed to tell them the real reason.

'And your phone? Is it sick too?' asked Mona sarcastically.

'I lost it,' she lied again, when in fact she had deliberately not answered their phone calls.

'Okay! Let's cheer you up,' said Shiela, and started telling a joke about a man whose wife said, '*Tum kal padosan ke saath movie dekhne gaye they* (Did you go to the movies with the lady next door yesterday)?'

The husband replied, '*Kya karun . . . aaj kal parivaar ke saath dekhne layak filme banti hi kahan hain?* (What to do, nowadays they don't make movies that can be watched with families)!'

Meera smiled weakly. She wouldn't dare laugh.

'You have lost your ability to laugh too!' lamented Shiela.

'No, I have lost my bladder control,' Meera blurted out.

'What?' Shiela and Mona exclaimed in unison.

The dam broke and the entire story came tumbling out, along with a torrent of tears.

Meera was now pouring her heart out, 'What was worse was what happened at the wedding we attended some time ago. I was in urgent need of visiting the loo but there were long lines in front of all the five toilet doors at the five-star hotel. My bladder was ready to burst but I knew I would have to wait. To my horror, I began to wet my silk salwar right there, like a baby! Thankfully, most of the women were engrossed in conversation and paid little attention to me. I backed against a wall and stood there, still as a statue, till the toilet nearest to me fell vacant, and rushed to lock myself in. I dared not come out in such a state and stayed in that cubbyhole for an hour! My husband did not notice my absence as he was busy drinking with his friends! It was that kind of wedding, where men get together around the bar and women daintily sip Sprite mixed with gin and tonic, all the while pretending to be *sati-savitris* who don't know what alcohol is!'

'Well, you certainly haven't lost *your* sense of humour!' said Mona with a small laugh.

'When did you finally come out?' asked Shiela, more interested in the outcome of this debacle.

'When I was reasonably sure that the ladies washroom was empty, I rang up my husband and told him about the mishap. I asked him to call the driver to the porch so that we would not have to wait for the car. Then I made him walk behind me to cover me in case there was a wet patch on my kurta, all the way till we reached the sanctuary of our vehicle, but worse was to follow.'

'Why, what happened?'

'You know our dog, Dusty; he suffers from motion sickness.'

'For God's sake, what has that to do with this?' exclaimed Shiela.

'The mystery is deepening,' said Mona with mock seriousness.

'*Yahan meri jaan pe ban aayi thi aur tujhe mazaak sujh raha hai* (It was a matter of life and death for me and you are making fun of me!)?' admonished Meera.

'Okay, carry on.'

'Well. We keep a rug in the boot for Dusty to sit on whenever we take him to the vet, so that he vomits on it and not on the car seat.'

'So?'

'My husband got the rug from the boot, placed it on the rear seat and made me sit on it while he sat in the front with the driver!'

'How could he?' exclaimed Mona, now feeling outraged.

'It was either this or an argument with my husband in front of the driver till we reached home,' Meera said with tears in her eyes. She had been deeply hurt and her friends could see that.

'Your husband is one mean bastard. I'll tell you what you should do: take his car keys one night when he is fast asleep and empty your bladder on his seat,' said the feminist Mona viciously.

'Thanks for your fierce loyalty, Mona, but though I was terribly hurt at that time, I now see things from his perspective. The smell of urine would remain till he got the car seat dry-cleaned or changed the upholstery, so it was better that I sat on a separate mat.'

'Has he changed his bed too?' Mona asked. There definitely was a faint smell of urine around their poor friend.

This was too painful a subject to discuss even with her closest friends. Shiela sensed her discomfiture and said, 'What have you done about it?

'I went to our GP for treatment.'

'And?'

'No concrete results. The test results were normal, though . . . I have reached the end of my patience. I felt like killing myself when my grandson said, "*Nani ko bhi diaper pehna do. Usse bhi* Gudiya *jaise sosoo ki smell aa rahi hai* (Make granny wear a diaper to. She too smells of urine, like Gudiya),"' said Meera, as a fresh bout of tears erupted from her eyes.

Shiela engulfed Meera in her arms and held her tight. It felt good to be comforted after months of agony. Meera cried her eyes out, and that melted somewhat the shards of icy pain that had grated upon her very soul.

'There, there now, stop crying,' soothed Mona. 'I'll take you to a gynaecologist.'

'A gynaecologist? Isn't this a kidney problem?' asked Meera. It never occurred to her to visit a gynaecologist. She had not been to one since her last childbirth.

'Could be, but more likely than not, it has something to do with menopause.'

'How do you know?'

'I have my sources,' said Mona mysteriously. 'A colleague had a similar problem, though in a milder form, and Dr Rosy worked wonders. I'll take you to her. Not only is she good at her job, she is also very compassionate and down-to-earth—so rare in doctors these days.'

'Is there really a treatment for it?' asked Meera in wonder. 'I thought that I was going to die of embarrassment!'

'Oh, come on, you'll be walking faster than Mona and me very soon!' Shiela comforted her.

'*Tere muh me ghee shakkar!* (I hope what you say is true),' said Meera, laughing for the first time in many days. Hope had been restored and there was nothing like hope to give a new lease of life, or a new lease to the quality of life, in her case.

An appointment was fixed and soon, Meera sat in a well-appointed waiting room. On the wall was hung a saying:

The patient will never care how much you know until they know how much you care.
—*Terry Canale*

This reassured Meera somewhat, as did the clasp of her friend's hand.

One look at the lovely doctor, with a twinkle in her eye and a sprig of jasmine in her hair, and Meera was won over. An immediate bond of trust was established between the two. Patiently, she heard Meera out and made her cough while examining her to check for what she called 'stress incontinence'. She asked her to get an uroflowmetry done.

This, the doctor explained, would differentiate between stress incontinence (leaking on straining) and urge incontinence (inability to hold urine), which, in turn would help her manage things. The former needed an operation while the latter could be treated with medicines. Women could have either or both. As it turned out later, Meera had both.

'In either case, your bladder control will be restored, and along with it your self-esteem,' concluded Dr Rosy.

'How well she understands a patient's psyche,' marvelled Meera.

By the end of the session, there had developed such a rapport between the two that the doctor confided, 'I too had urge incontinence (the "had" gave hope to Meera) and assumed it was a natural part of ageing that I would learn to live with. Gradually, the condition worsened. One night, I was unable to sleep after an emergency call and got up almost every hour to pee. Tired and unrefreshed, I made my way to the hospital in a bad mood. To my dismay, the first patient I saw in the OPD had symptoms exactly like mine! As she listed the same complaints that *I* was experiencing, I empathized with her. Even as I taught her to train her bladder by withholding her urine for at least five minutes more, whenever she felt the desire to urinate, my words sounded hollow to my ears. This exercise had not helped me at all. In fact, I felt a strong urge to pass urine myself that very instance. I made a beeline for the toilet soon after she left, only to be stopped by a medical representative who wanted to tell me about a new drug for urge incontinence in the market. The irony of the situation was that had I waited a moment longer, *my* urge would have made me incontinent right in front of him! I shooed him away and with my thighs pressed tightly together, taking small, stiff steps, I just about made it to the washroom.'

Meera found herself laughing with abandon for the first time in weeks. Here was a kindred soul who knew exactly what she was going through!

'Now, coming down to the nitty-gritty—the depletion of hormones after menopause affects not only the genital tract, but also the base of the bladder, leading to urinary problems. To rectify this deficiency, I am prescribing an oestrogen cream that you must insert in your vagina biweekly at night for three months. This will help restore the genitourinary system to its premenopausal state and decrease the urinary and sexual problems, if any, occurring due to vaginal dryness.'

The doctor had inadvertently solved another problem that Meera was reluctant to reveal, lest she be ridiculed for desiring sex at this age. Though the urinary leak worsened the situation, the excruciating pain due to vaginal dryness had forced her to stay away from sex. Hopefully, the operation and the cream would restore their sexual equilibrium. It was something she looked forward to and would surprise her husband on his birthday by taking the lead. Such pleasant thoughts brought a smile to her lips, but suddenly, she was scared.

'You are sure the operation will work, doctor?' she asked.

'It does give satisfying results,' the doctor replied. 'Stress incontinence occurs due to defects in the genito-urinary support system. It happens usually after trauma during childbirth but becomes an issue when tissues weaken at this age. This surgery reinforces the damaged tissue with a mesh that gives the support required. It takes only about fifteen minutes to half an hour. The mesh is expensive, though.'

'Anything, doctor, to improve the quality of my life,' said the distraught woman.

Three months and a small operation later, as Shiela had predicted, Meera was walking ahead with remarkable self-assurance. The shame and horror were fading memories. Gone was the weepy woman with a smell of urine about her. Around her now was the fragrance of flowers. So taken up was she by her doctor that she too had started wearing flowers in her hair. On her finger, she flaunted a diamond ring that her husband had given her on *his* birthday as a return gift for the surprise *she* had given him on satin bedsheets clad in sheer, black lingerie—a delightful secret that she would not share even with her dear friends.

> **Friendly advice:** It's important to get proper medical attention and follow medical advice if the quality of your life is being affected.

4

DO YOU STILL HAVE SEX?

Mona and her office friends had so enjoyed the session with Dr Rosy that they decided to make it a monthly affair. As for Pushpa, she literally worshipped the ground on which the doctor walked—her self-esteem and good humour had returned with the cessation of her symptoms, as had her work performance. Hot flashes and cold sweats were distant memories now. Today, they had all gathered to discuss a taboo subject, nonetheless exciting for it being forbidden: sex after menopause. Unlike the previous session, when they were wary of each other and also wondered what the doctor would say, today they were chatting away, eager to know all there was to know about 'it'.

Dr Rosy came dressed in a lavender, Lucknowi chikan saree with the trademark flower in her curls and an irrepressible smile on her lips. She looked at the eager group and said, 'You naughty girls!' at which they burst out laughing. They all knew the subject they were going to talk about. 'I am glad that you all are so keen to know about sex even at this age because the other day, I was addressing a group of middle-aged women medicos on this subject and was surprised at the number of doctors (other than gynaecologists)—sonographists, pathologists, dentists, physiotherapists—who flocked around me after the session, posing private queries pertaining to their sex lives. Many of them had been suffering silently for years and were keen on making up for lost time! If this was the state of my colleagues, I can well imagine what the other educated females, despite easy access to the internet (which, incidentally, one should *not* consult in medical matters), must be going through.

'I thought of women like you, corporate heads and other successful senior females in various fields, who were missing out on this major aspect of living because they were ignorant of the facts and shy about asking. They had become resigned to a life without intimacy, assuming it was a natural part of menopause.

'I hope to sweep the cobwebs of confusion from your minds and lead those who have strayed into arid wastelands back to bowers of sweet nectar. Forgive the flowery language, for I cannot take the writer out of me to give a dry talk on such a luscious subject, but a satisfying sex life in the autumn of life is worth investing in. Nothing can beat the afterglow, the relaxation, the sense of well-being and the improved interpersonal relationship. To love and want, to feel loved and wanted in return, will make you feel happy and young even at this age and, menopause will be just a blurry milestone that whizzes past in this heady journey towards self-fulfilment. When you are replete with pleasure and peace, there will be a glow on your face, a shine in your eyes that no beauty parlour can give. This will give a fillip to your self-confidence. Will it not?'

'Yes!' they all agreed, losing more of their inhibitions, as Dr Rosy had intended all along.

'I will not use the phrase "even at this age" again for it used to bug me when people said "We marvel at your zest for life even as this age" or "Your productivity is remarkable, even at this age" or "I would consider myself fortunate if I was half as active as you, even as this age". At one point, I had finally had enough of it and retorted, "What do you mean by 'even at this age'?" which shut them up once and for all! As I read somewhere, "age matters only if you are cheese, wine or scotch" and that is something we all must bear in mind. You are as young as you feel and fanning the fires of your sexuality will only add vibrancy to your life. I know that the corporate work squeezes you dry and you have neither the time nor the inclination for anything else but sleep, but you have to make an effort to revive and maintain your sex life as it is important for your well-being. How about a long, satisfactory Saturday night session when you can get up late the next day or a lazy Sunday afternoon? According to (Mishneh Torah, Hilkhot Shabbat 30:14,) it is a religious recommendation that a Jewish "husband and wife have sex on Shabbat, as this is considered part of the Shabbat delight" even if she is menopausal. How wonderful it would be if we could practise it too.'

'Yes,' said Rita. 'But on weekends, my husband reads the newspapers and watches TV all day long while he wants me to cook special meals to make up for the hurriedly cooked lunches and dinners on other days.'

'How about reading good books on sexual stimulation and satisfaction and surprising him with that sort of "making up" one night?' the doctor responded. 'You might find him helping you in the kitchen so that you two can get to bed early! It is rumoured that King Edward the VIII abdicated his throne for the twice married, twice divorced Mrs Wallis, for she had attained mastery in this art during a visit to China. We have the *Kama Sutra* to our credit, though personally, I think many of the convoluted postures shown are more acrobatics than sex.'

'Yes,' said a voice from the back while the others laughed. Dr Rosy felt good when people laughed at her jokes and with this group of intellectuals, she felt particularly happy.

'What we must also understand is that a woman's sexual response to her partner is related to her feelings for him, the quality of their relationship and her partner's age and health, which means that sexual dysfunction can be multifactorial and the situation is not going to change dramatically for the better after menopause. Like that story of the man who went to a doctor for glasses and was assured that he would be able read once his vision improved—nothing of that sort happened because the poor man did not know how to read! Similarly, menopause, though conducive to sexual freedom, will not help a marriage where a sexual rapport never existed in the first place. The situation can change only if both partners are willing to make a conscious effort to improve their relationship or visit a marriage counsellor, which most couples are unwilling to do at this stage of their lives.'

'What about those with no husband?' a scribbled note without a signature was passed from hand to hand till it reached Dr Rosy.

'Good question,' said Dr Rosy. 'Yes, what about a woman with normal sexual desire but no partner? I too fall in this group as my husband expired some years ago.'

The women looked at each other, marvelling at the way Rosy could become one of them, even as she retained the role of a teacher.

'Be it death, divorce, spinsterhood, a partner who is unable to perform or an insensitive partner who takes his pleasure but gives none in return—many circumstances may leave a woman in a lurch, sexually,' continued Dr Rosy.

'And pray what should they do?' asked the questioner, who was emboldened by Dr Rosy's candour and felt she could speak openly.

'They need to take matters into their own hands—literally and figuratively. There is nothing shameful or sinful about self-gratification. Someone recounted a hilarious incident that occurred in a five-star hotel. He was the duty manager there that night. Early in the morning, he was called by the housekeeping staff to have a look at a "pink object" that a guest had forgotten in her room's safe. The pink object turned out to be a dildo (a sex toy) so large that it was bent at the tip in the small safe! Even as they were examining the pink object, it began to vibrate! Not only had she forgotten to take it along, she had forgotten to switch it off too! Perhaps she had to put it away in a hurry. The lady in question was a very important guest, the CEO of a company that gave them a lot of business. She had married late but her loyalty to her "first partner" (the sex toy) remained because it had served her well on lonely business tours. A flurry of mails flew thick and fast between the guest and the hotel. She was asked if they should ship the pink object to her address. Horrified at the thought of her new husband receiving it in her absence, she asked them to dispose it off asap. This was done and of course, the privacy of the guest was strictly maintained.'

The house was in splits and Dr Rosy ended this little anecdote by saying, 'All of us may not have access to, or the inclination for, such gadgets, but there were other ways and means. Also, a caring husband who is unable to perform due to varying reasons like illness, decreased libido or erectile dysfunction can satisfy a wife with normal sexual desires, but in other ways.'

The girls were enjoying themselves thoroughly and eagerly waited for more. Dr Rosy did not disappoint them, for she said, 'After my husband expired, a cousin from the US was coming to India for a short holiday and rang up to ask if there was something I wanted from there. I politely refused her offer.

'"*Soch lo* Didi," she said, "I was thinking in terms of a vibrator."

'"What?" I asked, horrified and thrilled at the same time, but recovered my composure soon enough to say,

'"Thanks, but no thanks."

'"Why?"

'"I wouldn't be caught dead with it," I said, and then added, "Alive, I wouldn't mind it at all."

'"What do you mean?"

'"I am curious to see what it looks like and how it works but I dread the idea of my children finding it in my bedroom after my death."

'Sadly, no matter how mature they become, children never come to terms with their parents' sexuality. As for seeing how a vibrator looks and how it pleasures a woman, I finally got my wish while watching the movie *Lust Stories*. The female lead, in the last of the four stories (the one directed by Karan Johar) tries using it because her husband suffered from premature ejaculation and would leave her high and dry after each sexual encounter.'

When the laughter subsided, Dr Rosy continued, 'Now let's get down to some serious business. At the outset, I would like to say that there are women, be it due to cultural conditioning or religious restrictions (that propagate the view that sex is for procreation and not recreation), who prefer to abstain from sex during this period of life and it is entirely their choice.'

Roma, who wore a *rudraksh* mala around her neck, nodded in affirmation.

'If both partners are comfortable without sexual activity at this stage of their lives, it is their prerogative, but they should not be averse to kissing, cuddling or expressing their affection in little ways so that a loving relationship is maintained. I am now going to tell you a naughty joke in this context,' said Dr Rosy, her eyes twinkling with merriment. 'A grandson once asked his grandfather if he still had sex with his wife (the grandmother) and was surprised to hear that they were sexually active.

'Amazed at his grandfather's prowess, he cheekily asked, "How do you like it best?"

'"Oral."

'"Oral sex!"

'"Yes. Before going to bed, I tell her 'I f***k you' and she says the same to me before we go to sleep!"'

'A fine sense of humour the couple had, I must say!' quipped Reena.

'True,' said Dr Rosy and continued, 'With the "celibate by choice" out of the way, let's get down to the various sexual situations that can arise at this age:

- ♦ Normal desire for sex in both partners and satisfactory sex—no issues, continue as before
- ♦ Normal desire but intercourse is painful

♦ Decreased or absent libido
♦ Increased libido

'Let's take up the above scenarios one by one.

Pain during intercourse

This is the commonest reason that puts women off sex during the menopausal-perimenopausal period. The decreasing levels of female sex hormones decrease the blood supply to the vagina and decrease lubrication of the vaginal wall. As a result, the vaginal lining loses its elasticity and sponginess, becoming thin and dry. This leads to

♦ Vaginal soreness
♦ Itching
♦ Pain on penetration
♦ Cuts in the vaginal orifice (vestibule)
♦ Friction within a dry vagina during intercourse, akin to the grating of live tissue, is sheer torture; the importance of slime, a word we often use in a derogatory manner, is now appreciated
♦ When acidic urine (there is increased frequency and pain during urination at menopause) falls repeatedly on the sore vaginal opening, the burning becomes excruciating
♦ The thin, dry vagina is less resistant to invading organisms, leading to inflammation and infection
♦ Years after menopause, the external and internal genitalia shrink, making penetration difficult; drugs have been tried for this condition but

can, on rare occasions, cause genital cancer and
heart disease

This is more than enough to put anyone off sex
completely, though paradoxically, the more sex one has, the
better is the lubrication. Many times, you may want to have
sex, but your body does not cooperate. Added to the physical
torture is the guilt of not being able to satisfy your partner,
who feels that *you* have lost interest in him. This leads to a
sad and lonely situation in bed. Remember that there is help
available and the situation can be rectified to your mutual
satisfaction. If the soreness is mild, try using water-based
lubricating creams like KY jelly. Apply it internally just
before intercourse. If that does not help, consult your doctor
regarding local application of an oestrogen cream that keeps
the vagina moist and elastic, decreases the burning and
itching and prevents infections.

Local creams are organ-specific and are therefore safer
than oral hormonal preparations, which also act on other
systems and may have undesirable side effects. Even so,
oestrogen creams must be taken under medical supervision.'

'Everything clear so far? Shall I pause to take a few
questions? Better now, when they are fresh in your mind,
than at the end,' said Dr Rosy.

'I have read somewhere that keeping oneself hydrated
will prevent vaginal dryness,' said Mona. She already knew
the answer as she had talked about it personally with
Dr Rosy during a consult, but wanted her friends to benefit
from her advice too.

'False. "Read somewhere" or "googled it" is a bad
alternative to taking proper medical advice. The excess

water will be flushed out by the kidneys and does not permeate the vaginal wall. Moreover, it is not water but lubrication and elasticity that are needed. In fact, increased intake of water is harmful to people with kidney disease or heart failure.'

'Can we use Vaseline or face creams for lubrication?' asked Malvika.

'No. Oil-based lubricants like Vaseline provide a medium for bacterial growth, particularly in a person whose immune system has been weakened by chemotherapy or HIV infection or in those who are taking immunosuppressants after transplant surgery. They also weaken latex, the material used to make condoms.'

'Condoms during menopause?' asked Sheetal, amazed.

'Yes, you heard that right. Postmenopausal women need to use contraceptives for at least two years after the cessation of periods, as there can be erratic ovulation and you could end up becoming a mother instead of a grandmother! Moreover, condoms provide protection against STDs (sexually transmitted diseases) from a new or an unfaithful partner. In fact, one must be wary of new sexual partners at this age as the thin, dry vaginal mucosa is easily bruised and the chances of STDs increase manifold.'

'How do we use oestrogen creams?' asked Malvika, who would now have to stop using Vaseline.

'For that, you will have to come to the clinic for a consult as it is best used under medical supervision, but broadly speaking, 5 gm (as indicated on the applicator) has to be inserted high up in the vagina at bedtime every night for two weeks and biweekly for three months. Take a gap of a month or so after this and restart biweekly if symptoms recur.'

'Such a bother,' said Malvika. 'Might as well try KY jelly first.'

'KY jelly is good for mild cases but if dryness worsens with age, this is a wonderful option,' said Dr Rosy. 'Now, let's move on to the next group of women who would like to have sex but are unable to muster the interest.

Decreased libido

During menopause, the circulating levels of oestrogen decrease, reducing the desire for sex. Even if her partner does his best, the woman is not as easily aroused by foreplay, while those who have pain during sex develop a phobia and resist getting intimate. Her partner feels hurt by what he thinks is her loss of interest in him and loses interest due to her lack of interest, which finally leads to abstinence and an unfortunate situation in bed.

Those with high-profile jobs and increased stress levels like yours and mine are too tired and all they want to do in bed is sleep. At this stage, it would be a good idea to leave the kids with their grandparents or other family members and take a break "far from the madding crowd" so that you can rediscover each other (and that includes your erotic zones) and come back with your interest in love and sex rejuvenated. Since not everyone can spare the time for a vacation or have grannies to look after the children, I suggest you keep some part of the weekend for yourselves—find ways of spending time together. However, other factors that can also contribute to a decreased libido are:

◆ Poor bladder control: the repeated visits to the toilet after sex can put her off sex, and the faint

smell of urine about the woman, can put off her partner
- Sleep disturbances
- Psychological issues such as stress, depression, anxiety
- Side effect of medications taken for other conditions
- Systemic illnesses: like diabetes, hypertension, psychiatric illnesses, anaemia

If a woman is distressed over her lack of sexual desire or her partner is distressed over *her* lack of sexual desire, there are means to improve it. These include:

- Remedial measures listed above for dry vagina, if that is the cause
- HRT: replacement of oestrogen helps in regaining
- libido
- If there are side effects with oestrogen, a drug called Tibilone can be used
- Testosterone patches are being tried abroad for decreased libido but can lead to Masculinization (fascial hair, hoarseness of voice and other masculine manifestation in females)

Please note that HRT should be taken strictly under medical supervision after a battery of tests, and that too only if the benefits outweigh the risks. Rigorous follow-up is mandatory as it can have severe side effects at times, like breast cancer and endometrial cancer (cancer of the inner lining of the womb).

Increased sexual drive

Some postmenopausal women experience increased sex drive. To understand the reason, you must know that all females have a small amount of testosterone in their blood, which is responsible for their libido. Due to the decreased levels of female hormones, the little testosterone we have in our blood gets the upper hand and improves sex drive. It is also responsible for postmenopausal hirsutism. Like a gynaecologist once said, the husband of a hairy woman told her, '*Tum mujhe aise nahin achhi lagti magar waise achhi lagti ho* (I don't like you like this but I like you like that).' What he meant was that though the facial hair put him off, her taking the initiative during sex turned him on!

Other factors that contribute to increased sex desire are:

♦ Fewer or no child-rearing responsibilities
♦ Relaxed atmosphere, retired husband, utter privacy and all the time in the world
♦ No fear of unwanted pregnancy
♦ No need for contraception (except for the first two years)

'What advice do I give these women? Nothing: just enjoy yourself if your partner is up to the new you!'

Never had the girls enjoyed a 'talk' so much, but Dr Rosy had not finished yet.

'Once, a forty-two-year-old woman came to me for tightening of her vagina as there was no sensation during intercourse.

'"Here comes another one," I thought, fuming inwardly. The husband of my previous patient had incited my feminist anger by wanting to know the sex of their child. "We already have a daughter, so why would we want another?" he'd explained, as reasonably as he could to a moron like me!

'"I don't know about that, but I do know what I can do with you—send you to jail!" I said through clenched teeth and showed them the door. So when the next patient came, I was already on the edge. "Tell your husband that your vagina has become lax delivering *his* children," I told her.

'After a moment of stunned silence, she said, "*I* can't feel anything going inside."

'Covering my embarrassment at being so vocal about imaginary MCPs, I said gently, "Oh, there is an operation to tighten a loose vagina." She eventually didn't get the surgery done but that is beside the point. Sigh. I could write a book on the things I see every day,' said Dr Rosy. 'The very next day, there was another extreme case. A forty-five-year-old woman came to the free OPD I go to once a week. She was distressed because her husband had been forcing himself on her without respite for years. "Then why are you coming to me now?" I asked and learnt that since she had attained menopause, the friction within her dry vagina night after night was sheer torture. "He is a sick man," I told her and asked her to either get rid of his mental issues or get rid of him. But such things are easier said than done. Being from an economically poor background with no income of her own, she could not go back to her poor parents. Her husband earned enough from his tiny general store in the front room of their home (from where he aimed missiles of invective towards her between serving customers) to take care of the household expenses and the children's education. When she gave her mother a hint of her problem, she was told that it was the wife's duty to take care of her husband's needs, whether she liked it or not! Indeed! She tried confiding in a friend who, she was amazed to learn, was actually envious of her and sighed, "My husband can barely get it up; I would gladly exchange places with you!"

'All I could suggest was to take him to a psychiatrist, but I knew that this was one horse that would not even go to the "water", leave alone drink it. The poor woman left the clinic dejected for I could do nothing to help her.'

To break the quiet that had suddenly descended in the room, Dr Rosy asked, trying to change the atmosphere, 'So what is your take-home message regarding intimacy in the postmenopausal period?'

'Remain sexually active for as long as you can,' said Mona.

Rosy gave her a thumbs-up and repeated, 'Remain sexually active for an increased sense of wellbeing and improved interpersonal relationship. It also increases the blood flow to the vagina and aids lubrication which makes intercourse a pleasurable affair instead of a painful one.

Needless to say, the applause was thunderous after it was all over.

Friendly advice: Sexual intimacy is as relevant in the post-menopausal period as it was earlier; issues that arise due to decreased hormone levels can be dealt with by seeking medical help.

5

A BABY AT THIS AGE!

Mona and Rita were the best of friends at their office, Mascot Enterprises. On account of the cut-throat competition, colleagues in a corporate firm could not be 'real' friends, but these two got along tolerably well. They shared stories of corporate politics, and vented their frustrations about unreasonable bosses, impossible deadlines and flirtatious creeps, which Mona's dear colony friends Shiela and Meera would never understand. And now, coincidentally, both missed their period—Mona was forty years old and Rita forty-two! Being smart office heads, keenly aware of how they carried themselves, both wondered if they had attained premature menopause; it would definitely undermine their confidence. They also knew that there was nothing they could do about it. Neither even dreamt that she could be pregnant. Mona had been childless for so long despite fertility treatments that the thought did not even occur to her. As for Rita, she was so busy managing her home, her career and her two boisterous teenage boys that she hardly had time for sex.

What Mona did realize was that her appetite had decreased considerably over the previous two weeks. She pecked at her food in the office canteen while Rita urged her to eat. When she was so revolted by her favourite Chinese meal that she got up to vomit, it struck Rita that Mona could be pregnant. After all, she had given birth to two children herself and knew the signs. When Mona returned from the toilet, looking wan and sick, Rita made her relax and sip some coconut water. Only when the colour returned to her cheeks did Rita ask, 'Have you got a pregnancy test done?'

'Why on earth should I? I have never conceived before despite treatment.'

'There is always a first time. Test your urine first thing tomorrow morning.'

A thrill of joy and apprehension coursed down Mona's spine. 'Could it really be true? Had the Almighty finally showered His benevolence on her? But a child at this age?' A hundred different thoughts raced through her mind, flitting across her expressive face like a play of the sun and clouds on a clear blue sky. She was excited and terrified at the same time. Her emotions were reflected on her face in the form of a shy smile and a blush, and then a frown. Rita watched, fascinated, till it struck her that *she* had better practice what she preached. She had never missed her periods and though sexual encounters in her marital life were few and far between, there was always a chance.

So both friends took a pregnancy test kit back home and met the next morning with the results. Both were pregnant, but their reaction was as different as day from night.

Mona was as radiant as the moon, and Rita was as gloomy as the night. Mona rang up Dr Rosy and asked her to see them. They needed her advice urgently.

'I'll see if there are any cancellations in my OPD schedule; is it an emergency?' asked Dr Rosy, concerned.

'Yes,' Mona said for the both of them, though they both had different reasons.

'I'll try to squeeze you in,' said Dr Rosy.

'We are coming,' announced Mona with finality and ended the call. Dr Rosy looked at the phone in her hand, shaking her head with an amused smile.

'This girl is impossible,' she said to herself, but Mona had become a dear friend and she could not refuse her.

Finally, the two were seated in her office and Dr Rosy realized that their 'emergency' was not of the medical kind. Both were in the perimenopausal period, and both were pregnant! Mona was ecstatic while Rita was glum. Mona wanted to keep the pregnancy at all costs and Rita wanted to get rid of it as soon as possible. A doctor is but an instrument in the hands of her patients, catering to their needs provided it is medically safe and legal. In a single day, a doctor sees a patient desperate for a child, another begging her to get rid of it and a third in the throes of labour.

As a consult is confidential and their requirements were different, Dr Rosy knew where to draw the line. The privacy of a patient was of prime importance; even the best of friends would not like to reveal intimate details of their lives in front of each other. They would readily trust the secrets of their minds and bodies with their doctor, which imposes a great responsibility on this noble profession.

Realizing the seriousness of the situation, she attended to Rita first.

'So Rita, are you sure that you do not want to continue with this pregnancy?'

'There is no doubt about that. I already have two grown-up sons,' said Rita emphatically.

'Normal deliveries?'

'No, both caesareans.'

'Any abortions?'

'Yes, one, soon after the birth of my second son, but it was so early that MTP pills sufficed.'

'Were you using any contraception?'

'No. We hardly do it. Who would have thought I would conceive at this age?'

'And yet here you are.'

'Yes, here I am. Now what?'

'I'll examine you internally, get an ultrasound done to confirm the exact age of your pregnancy, and depending upon that, we'll decide on the method of termination. When did you have your last period?'

'About two, two and a half months back.'

'You don't remember exactly when?'

'No, I did not feel the need to monitor them at this age.'

Dr Rosy let that pass; instead, she asked, 'Were your periods regular?'

'Yes.'

'It didn't occur to you that you may be pregnant?'

'No. I thought it was menopause.'

'Do you know that women can get pregnant till two years after they have stopped menstruating?'

'How can they?'

'Erratic ovulation does occur once in a while, and usually women get to know that they are pregnant only after the baby starts moving and can do nothing else but deliver it. *Budhape ki aulad* (a child of old age), as they used to say in the olden days. My *nani* did not have a single period after she started having babies because she would conceive her next child while feeding her newborn. There is but a difference of a year or two between my uncles and aunts. Well, no point in discussing all that now. Get the ultrasound report and we will decide accordingly.'

Rita returned the next day with her husband Rohan Rathi and the report, which showed a nine-week-old foetus. The termination would have to be a surgical procedure in the OT under anaesthesia.

'Anything you say, doctor, as long as she is safe,' said Rohan.

'Another thing I want to ask you both is about contraception. I can insert an intrauterine contraceptive device (IUCD) in the same sitting, if you agree—of course, after I explain the pros and cons to you.'

'No thanks, doctor!' said Rita vehemently. 'I have experienced only the cons of an IUCD.'

'What do you mean?'

'I was persuaded to get it inserted after my first child but after a year of heavy, painful periods I got rid of it. There is a gap of just two years between my two boys. Also, a friend became pregnant with the IUCD in place, so what's the use?'

'Every contraceptive, for that matter every allopathic medicine has some side effect which is usually mild. Though IUCD is convenient and safe, I am sorry it did not work for you. I will definitely not "persuade" you to do anything against your wishes.'

'What other options do you have?'

'Well, there are contraceptive pills that have to be taken regularly but under strict medical supervision, especially at this age.'

'I am quite forgetful, so this option is not for me. Moreover, I am too lazy to visit a doctor unless something is really wrong with me.'

'As for withdrawal method, condoms . . .'

Before Dr Rosy could finish her sentence, Rita blurted out, 'Rohan says using a condom is like eating a toffee with the wrapper on!' embarrassing her husband who did not know where to look.

Dr Rosy smiled at the apt analogy and said, 'You did not let me complete my sentence. I was trying to tell you that these methods have a high failure rate and are not recommended at this age. That leaves us with just one option, the permanent one—tubal ligation. While under anaesthesia, a laparoscope is passed into your abdomen through a key hole, the tubes that carry the egg from the ovaries to the uterus are identified and blocked so that the sperm and eggs do not meet and conception does not occur. It is also called female sterilization.'

'I'll go for that,' said Rita with alacrity.

'It is a surgical procedure, and you must be aware that this too can fail, though it very rarely does.'

'I am willing to take the chance.'

'Why don't you discuss it with Rohan and get back to me later?'

'What is there to discuss?' said Rita. 'He doesn't have to go through all this.'

Dr Rosy looked questioningly at Rohan.

'I am okay with whatever she wants,' he said.

'We can get *you* vasectomized . . .' suggested Dr Rosy tentatively.

Again, Rita intervened forcefully, 'What's the need? I am getting anesthetized anyway, so let's concentrate on me.'

Dr Rosy was aware of the misconception that vasectomy

decreased masculine potency, hence the reluctance, but this is not the time to discuss that. Moreover, as Rita rightly pointed our she was getting anesthetized anyways; might as well tie her tubes.

Both the procedures were soon performed successfully and a very satisfied Rita left the hospital the next day.

Mona was a completely different case altogether.

'So, Mona, how are you feeling?' asked Dr Rosy.

'Elated.'

'You want to keep the pregnancy.'

'As close to my heart as possible.'

'Cut out the dramatics and tell me, why haven't you brought your husband along?' asked Dr Rosy with a smile.

'He is away on a business tour and I am hugging the delicious secret to myself. He will be returning on the eve of our fifteenth anniversary. I'm sure he'll bring me a lovely gift from Singapore, but for the first time in all these years, *my* gift will be better; the best!'

'True,' agreed Dr Rosy. 'Now show me your ultrasound report.'

Dr Rosy saw a six-week pregnancy with a robust heart rate sitting snug in the uterus and said, 'All good.'

'That's all you've got to say?' Mona took the liberty of asking, for the two had become fast friends over time.

'And will you frame and hang the first photograph of your "bean-like" baby in your drawing room?'

'Yes!' laughed Mona, too happy to contain her joy.

'Now, calm down and let's revert to the doctor-patient relationship or I'll have to refer you to a colleague.'

'Over my dead body,' said Mona, suddenly serious.

'*Shubh shubh bolo* (Say only auspicious things). I want you to know that we need to be cautious about pregnancies in the forties. They are called by such demoralizing names as "geriatric pregnancy" or "elderly primi", and fall in the high-risk category.'

'Risks? I'm scared,' said Mona, swinging from one end of the pendulum to the other. 'I don't want anything to happen to my baby.' Stress was definitely not good for her.

'I don't want anything to happen to *you* and your baby, understood?' said Dr Rosy, adding, 'The good news is that more and more women are opting for late pregnancy due to work, late marriage, infertility and IVF pregnancy (the number has more than doubled over the years) and are doing very well. Some of the celebrities I could name are Meghan Markle, Julia Roberts . . .'

Mona brightened visibly because the ladies mentioned were enjoying their motherhood with healthy children; in fact, Julia Roberts had twins!

'To think that I had given up trying to conceive a long time ago when the fertility guy suggested the use of donor eggs, and now this windfall!'

'You were not able to conceive probably because you were trying too hard.'

'You are absolutely right. I did not want a baby for years, till I was "settled" in my career, and when I wanted one, I wanted it instantly.'

'Like two-minute noodles. That is not how Mother Nature works. Well, she has forgiven you and gifted a baby to your womb. It is up to us, you and me, to nurture it to the best of our ability.'

'So how do we go about it?'

'I want you to understand once and for all that, stress will be counterproductive. You are very high-strung, so please learn relaxation techniques like pranayama and meditation and practice them diligently.'

'Okay.'

'Now, let's get down to business. We have made an excellent start by having a natural conception, but there is still a long, hazardous way to go.'

'What do you mean?'

'There are risks peculiar to a pregnancy this late in life, the most scary being a baby with Down syndrome or other chromosomal abnormalities.'

'What is Down's Syndrome?'

'It is a form of mental retardation due to genetic abnormalities.'

'OMG!' said Mona with a shudder.

'God, please God, let my baby be healthy and normal,' she prayed silently.

And that was not all. She listened with increasing alarm as Dr Rosy listed the risks associated with increasing maternal age:

♦ **Gestational diabetes:** diabetes may pre-exist or become overt for the first time during pregnancy, and may or may not continue after delivery. It complicates the pregnancy in various ways, is detrimental to foetal health and may even cause intrauterine foetal demise. Moreover, those who have gestational diabetes may develop diabetes later in life.

♦ Hypertension: high blood pressure may pre-exist or become overt for the first time during pregnancy, and may or may not continue after delivery. If the woman also has albumin in her urine, the condition is called preeclampsia, which can have a detrimental effect on the pregnancy. Those who have gestation hypertension or preeclampsia may develop hypertension in later life.

- Down syndrome or other chromosomal abnormalities in the child, as already mentioned.
- Miscarriages are common as the quality of the egg deteriorates at this age and there may be chromosomal abnormalities incompatible with life.
- IUGR: intrauterine growth-restricted babies, which may be unexplained or due to hypertension, diabetes etc.
- Preterm delivery for which the baby needs admission in the nursery and may be exposed to hospital infections.
- Low birth weight due to IUGR
- Placental issues: placental insufficiency which means that the placenta does not function optimally and is unable to supply adequate amount of oxygen and nutrients to the baby, impeding its growth; some pregnancies may be complicated by a dangerous condition called placenta previa, when the placenta is situated lower than the baby which can lead to life-threatening bleeding.
- Stillbirth: there is a slightly higher chance of the baby being born dead.
- Caesarean sections the chance of having an operative delivery increases with advancing age.
- Past medical history (medical problems increase with increasing age), family history of medical

issues and genetic abnormalities also impact the pregnancy in a negative way.

'Oh my God!' exclaimed Mona, looking at her with stricken eyes. 'You have frightened me out of my wits.'

'I hope your effervescence has subsided somewhat,' said Dr Rosy, for at times one had to be cruel to be kind. Unable to sustain her brutal stance for long, Dr Rosy laid a hand on Mona's shoulder and said kindly, 'Only *some* women over the age of thirty-five with a pregnancy experience some of the above complications, some of the time. You have conceived naturally, you are fit, active physically and mentally, your weight is optimal and you have no pre-existing medical conditions, so there is no reason why you should not have an easy pregnancy and delivery.' She noticed with satisfaction that the cloud on Mona's face had lifted to reveal a sunny smile, though just how easy her pregnancy and delivery would be, even Dr Rosy had not anticipated at that time.

'Now let me tell you some of the positives of a later age pregnancy,' said Dr Rosy. 'You will age later, have lower chances of getting Alzheimer's and live longer as you have so much child-rearing in the years ahead to live for. However, the bottom line is that there are no guarantees in life, and if you are willing to take the chance after being fully aware of the difficulties you may encounter, I am with you all the way. Even if you do get gestational diabetes and hypertension, I am sure it will be mild and I am there to take care of it.'

'Thank you, doctor, but I am most worried about Down's Syndrome. Can we know for sure before the birth of the baby?'

'Off course.'

'How?'

'Tests like NIPS (Non-invasive prenatal testing), amniocentesis and CVS (chorionic villus sampling) confirm or rule out the condition.'

'And it the report is positive . . . then what?'

'As it can be diagnosed early in pregnancy, when MTP (Medical termination of pregnancy) is legal, one can opt for an abortion.'

Thankfully Mona's reports were negative for Down's Syndrome. We leave her here for the time being, in the capable hands of Dr Rosy. She goes for regular antenatal follow ups, is particular about her medicines and exercise regimen though, with her volatile nature she is given to bouts of ecstasy alternating with apprehension, which, the good doctor knows very well how to handle.

6

IS IT TOO LATE FOR ROMANCE?

Dr Rosy Dua, Rosy to her close ones, had invited a few of her girlfriends over for her fifty-sixth birthday. Her husband had died four years back and she had finally made peace with the void his absence had created. She looked resplendent in a pink chiffon sari and a pink rose tucked into her curls. There was an animated chatter and bonhomie as these high-profile women forgot their work-problems and let their hair down. Chetna was a happily married doctor of forty-five years and still enjoyed a healthy sex life. She could not imagine living without a man and wondered how Rosy was faring all alone. Out of the blue she blurted, 'Its high time you brought some joy back in your life, Dr Rosy.'

'Whatever gave you the idea that I am unhappy?' countered Rosy.

'You still have a long active healthy life ahead of you. You are pretty, intelligent, look no older than forty . . .'

'So, what do you want me to do?'

'Add some romance to your life, *yaar.*'

The others stopped talking, intrigued by the turn the conversation had taken.

'Isn't it a bit too late for romance?' asked Dr Rosy, uncertainly.

'Certainly not!' interposed Sujata, a fifty-year-old divorcee with a son, who was studying abroad. Unable to bear the loneliness she was secretly looking at the app 'Second Chance' that introduced spinsters/bachelors, widows/widowers and divorcees seeking partners to each other.

'Then why haven't *you* got hitched again?' asked Dr Rosy.

'It's not for want for trying. For all you know, you may hear the news of my remarriage soon!'

'Really!!!' all were agog with excitement.

'Good for you,' sighed Mansi a forty-eight-year-old spinster, who had been so busy bringing up her siblings after her father's untimely death that she felt that she had missed the marital boat.

'I can help you find a partner too,' said Sujata, sensing Mansi's sadness. 'Let's talk in private later, I will tell you how to go about it,' Sujata whispered in her ear. Mansi's face lit up at the prospect.

Chetna clapped her hands to grab their attention once again and said 'We are straying from the subject. Let me tell you, Rosy,' she said. 'If you had died, no matter how much your husband loved you, he would have married again by now. Why haven't you?'

Dr Rosy said nothing but realized that she was living in a state of denial all this while. Occasionally, a wave of acute longing would rise that crashed against the wall of 'propriety' that she had built around her emotions. It was bound to crack one day.

'Rosy, we are still waiting for an answer?'

'*Log kya kahenge* (What will people say)?'

'I would like to ask you what these *log*, the *thekedaars* (caretakers) of society, did for you? Except for lip service in the initial days of bereavement not one walked that extra mile with you, on the long, lonely road ahead,' countered Naina, joining the conversation. 'You know what,' she continued animatedly. '*I* got my brother-in-law, a seventy-year-old widower married to my school-friend, a fifty-year-old spinster, and both are living happily together.'

'That was very of nice you.'

'Cut off this polite nonsense and listen to me, Rosy,' said Naina. 'By this age most of us have braved life's bumps, big and small and emerged stronger. We have lived long enough to know what exactly we want from life. So, if you really feel the need for a partner or have found one who complements you, hold on to him. To hell with societal norms!'

Dr Rosy could not agree more with this sentiment. With her children grown up and gone, she often experienced moments of utter loneliness and complete isolation. Unlike other widows, who turned to religion, kitty parties and beauty parlours, she had no interest in such pursuits. She did have a career to keep her busy, but returned to an empty house at the end of the day. With no one to share a thought, a meal, a bed and a home; no one to console her when she was feeling low and no one to cuddle up to for warmth, a sense of abandonment would overwhelm her. The modern mantra of 'positive thinking' with which she tried to numb herself, would go for a toss and bouts of self- pity would wash over her.

'But what about the children?' asked Dr Rosy, relenting a bit.

Surprisingly, the most vehement objections come from one's own children; the very offspring who have neither the time nor the inclination to give the attention and affection one craves. Yet, they resent the presence of another in one's life. Due to fear of the loss of their inheritance or public ridicule, they blackmail emotionally by saying things like, 'How could you forget Papa?'

It isn't as if one relationship was exclusive of the other and the presence of a new partner erased the memory of a previous loved one, but most women were not strong enough to brave the objections of the family and society. They end up suppressing their desires as they have been conditioned to do so all their lives. Children should be sensitive to the needs of a lonely parent instead of putting obstacles in their path; especially, if they are unable to do as much as they ought to for them. How can they expect a parent to mourn the dead all their lives; to throttle life out of living and merely exist? If the parents are expected to fend for themselves in all other aspects of living without their children's help, what gave them the right to put spokes in their wheel if they wish to fill the void in their life with a companion?

'All lot of children do understand their parent's plight. Remember Kajal? She was a resident with us a few years ago,' said Mansi. 'As the only child, she became the sole caretaker of her father after her mother's death. It became increasingly difficult for her to manage her profession, her young family and a father with diabetes, high blood pressure and angina. This led to absenteeism from work and poor performance, which her superiors did not take kindly to. Exasperated, she got her father married to a poor, distant relative, a forty-five-year-old widow with no children. The lady happily accepted the offer of a caretaker in exchange for a home of her own and a status in society.'

'That was not due to any altruistic motive but to shift her responsibility on another's shoulder; moreover, it's different for men,' murmured Dr Rosy.

'So says our fiery feminist!' mocked Mansi. 'For your information, Kajal's father married a widow. Even my neighbour, a timid, sheltered housewife is better than you. She jokingly told her husband that she would marry again as soon as he expired because she would not be able to manage the taxes, bills, etc. without a man!'

'A couple of years after my husband's death,' said Dr Rosy, 'my daughter-in-law said, "We haven't attended a marriage ceremony in ages. I would love to wear dressy clothes, heavy jewellery and dance the night away but there is no one of marriageable age in our family." Then, after a pause she came up with the bright idea of marrying me off! I was flummoxed. Of all the reasons to get married, this was the corniest. Though I laughed it off, I realized that there were times when loneliness mocked my façade of self-sufficiency. I was tempted to shock her by saying that I would indeed like a companion but out of wedlock (the very word suggested being in lockup). I had had enough of male dominance to last me a lifetime. A woman of my age living in "sin" was unthinkable in our regressive society so, I told her "I don't know about marriage, but I would love to travel the world and though I may appear to be a woman of the world, I am scared to do so alone." If only I could . . .' I said tentatively.

'And what did she say?' asked Sujata, curious.

'She said that there are escorts available for that, all over the world.'

'Who serve as gigolos too!' laughed Sujata.

Dr Rosy slapped her playfully on her thigh.

'Seriously, Dr Rosy, tell me if you have found someone but are too scared to follow it up. We are there to support you.'

'Well,' began Dr Rosy tentatively, 'I had gone for a class reunion some time ago. A motely bunch of men and women, previous classmates gathered at a beautiful resort in the middle of the lush forest. Here, we shed the cloak of age and felt as young and happy as we did during our college days. There were jungle safaris early in the mornings, gourmet meals, teasing banter and reminiscences. It was at night that we truly came alive—singing and dancing around a bonfire under a yellow January moon. A classmate, who had a soft corner for me during our college days, began to show an inordinate interest in me. He too had lost his spouse sometime back. Though I was not physically attracted to him, it felt nice to be desired. People began teasing us and I would blush like a schoolgirl. When he finally did propose, I refused. I knew that it was an honour and a privilege to be asked at all, at this age, but I realized sadly that both of us were too set in our ways and cities and it would be cruel to uproot one for the sake of the other. I held a senior post at a corporate hospital in Delhi and he was the Medical Superintendent of a private hospital in Nagpur. Moreover, if we married, we would also be marrying the ailments that come with age. Taking care of each other's debilities without knowing whether there would be happy years of togetherness in the future or not would have led to frustration. I wouldn't want to impose upon him my health issues that would eventually crop up as I aged, and I had enough of caring for the chronically ill to last me a lifetime. First, I looked after my mother-in-law through years of Alzheimer and hip fracture, then my husband through his terrible struggle with bladder cancer till he passed away and then there was my beloved aging little Lhasa Apso, Choco.

'Coming back to the reunion; on the last night of those magical days, we sat at a small table in the dining hall having our last meal together. The poignancy of the moment was beyond words. Our hearts were full though, I was mildly annoyed with him. He was fiddling with his cell phone, when he ought to be looking longingly into my eyes. I was mistaken. Soon enough he set the phone on the table and a beautiful, apt melody began to play softly:

'Lag ja gale, ke phir ye haseen raat ho na ho
Shayad phir is janam me mulakaat ho na ho'

(Let's embrace each other for there may never be a night as beautiful as this

We may never be able to meet again in this life).

'As if on cue we got up and embraced in a hall full of people. No one noticed! A crowd, I realized is the most private place in the world. I also realized that a warm, loving hug was welcome at any age and that the emotions it evoked were the same at all ages. It was never too late for romance. We still maintain contact and share each other's joys and sorrows on the phone and that is sufficient for me.'

Later, when Dr Rosy, discussed the subject of 'Love in Later Life' with the ladies of Mascot Enterprises, she concluded her talk by saying:

'Women, the world over, tend to outlive their male partners not only due to the age difference, but because they are the stronger sex in matters that really matter. They have the capacity of endurance (after all labour pains are one of the worst pains a human can endure) while all that, men can boast of, is brute strength. As a result, more and more women find themselves alone in the sunset period of their lives. Within their empty nests, a lot of these single women face complete isolation and utter loneliness. Having a partner at this age will not only improve the quality of their lives but will contribute majorly to longevity.

'The need for intimacy and emotional bonding exists at every stage of life. If she is embarrassed about her age and appearance as menopause does bring with it a bag of insecurities, remember that the person she is likely to meet is sailing in the same boat. It is the animated countenance, your conversational skills, a sense of humour and a helpful gesture attracts and endures more than your looks and figure. If there is a person whose company you enjoy, meet him over a cup of coffee or call him over for a quiet meal. To know that there is someone with whom you can talk about your day, share life events can bring great joy. A sympathetic ear, a kind word and a gentle touch will keep depression at bay. Such love need not always be consummated, and such interactions need not always end up in marriage.

'Don't let social stigma or self-reproach stop you from forming such relationships. Remember that you have the right to seek companionship. Memoires of your departed partner will not diminish if you grab moments of happiness with another. Let no one tell you otherwise and send you on a guilt trip.

'There is a beautiful story I read of an old man and woman. They were strangers, who sat on the same bench in a park after their evening walk. Gradually they got down to talking about their lives and their deceased spouses, whom they sorely missed. Eventually the two married with the understanding that each would be buried next to their original spouses after their deaths. This about sums up the ethos of a relationship in the second innings of life. I pictured the two watching the sunset from the same park bench, even after they were married and wrote:

> Let's sit together on our park bench
> As, with a contented sigh I put,
> My head on your shoulder while
> You hold my wrinkled hand in yours;
> And, in the quiet sunset of our lives
> Let's watch the sun, set over our day.
> Let dusk arrive to cloak our world with,
> The dusky colours of our twilight years.
> Let's wait awhile, to gaze in rapture
> At the moonless, star-studded night.
> But when the chill begins to bite let's
> Head homewards to our cosy cottage
> To thaw,
> The cold in our bones, by the fire
> The cold in our bellies, with steaming stew
> The cold in our lives, with warm hugs
> And lift joined hands heavenwards
> In a heartful prayer of gratitude for,
> The sweet companionship He granted us
> To navigate, the rest of our lives together.

7

THE RIVER FLOWED RED
AUB (Abnormal Uterine Bleeding)

Shiela could not keep pace with Meera and Mona during their evening walk. She had not been keeping well of late. Though she was fifty-three years of age, her periods hadn't stopped. In fact, they were more frequent and were heavier than before. While most women dreaded menopause, she longed to be free of the sanitary pads that she had to change every hour these days. They irritated her rather chubby inner thighs, which had become red and sore with friction while walking. Though she did not realize it, her haemoglobin levels were declining steadily. This made her irritable and snappy. Just the other day, she had been extremely harsh with a junior staff member, Mala, over a small mistake.

Mala could barely wait to vent. The moment she was out of the principal's room she said, 'I hate that bloody bitch. I hate her with all my heart. Why doesn't she just drop dead?'

'Lower your volume,' said her friend. 'I think principal ma'am has overheard.'

'I don't care,' she had said recklessly as she fiercely wiped away her tears.

Shiela was shocked by the outburst and was immediately repentant. She had indeed overreacted, but there was no way she could call the young teacher back and apologize. It would undermine her authority as principal of the nursery school she had run smoothly for over twenty-five years. She could do nothing but continued eavesdropping

'She must be going through *that* phase of her life,' consoled her friend.

'Whatever—she has no right to take her frustration out on someone who cannot retaliate.'

'If only the poor girl knew how sorry I am,' thought Shiela helplessly.

She did not know what had come over her, and it was the same at home. She snapped at her husband, servants and daughters-in-law. Though, her spouse bore her outbursts without retaliating (over the years he had learnt that silence was the best policy at such times), the servants quit and her daughters-in-law Rama and Reena told their husbands, through whom they retaliated. Life had become a mess and she did not know what to do. Her only solace was her evening walk with her friends but now, that too seemed like an impossible task.

This time her periods had started ten days earlier and would not stop. She was passing large clots that seemed to drain the very life out of her. She lagged behind her friends and was unable to keep pace with them. When she could not take a step further, she told the other two, 'You two continue. I think I'll go back home.'

Meera and Mona were walking ahead in animated conversation, little realizing that they had left Shiela behind. They turned to look at her pale, perspiring face and were alarmed. Quickly, they sat her down and gave her some water.

'What happened?'

'I have been passing large clots for the past ten days and am feeling totally drained.'

'Why didn't you visit a doctor?' demanded Meera.

'*Arre yaar*, it's the menopausal thing. Everyone says that the menstrual cycle becomes heavy and irregular towards the end. If only it would end. I am fed up.'

'You look absolutely pale. You must see a gynae at once. I'll fix an appointment for tomorrow,' said the efficient Mona, who was already looking on her phone for an empty a slot in Dr Rosy Dua's schedule.

'No,' said Shiela, but not vehemently enough. She had reached the end of her tether and was glad that someone else was taking charge for a change. After years of shouldering the responsibilities of her school and home, it felt good to be taken care of. Her husband and sons ran a chartered accountancy firm and as it was nearing the end of the financial year, they could not spare a minute. She had always made excuses for the men in her life, who had neglected her, and she felt her daughters-in-law had learnt from them—they too did not seem to care much. Shiela did not realize that she appeared so formidable and totally in control that no one had an inkling of the fact that she too needed attention and affection. As far as Rama and Reena were concerned, she was someone they had to steer clear of. Being a busy working woman Shiela had chosen nonworking wives for her sons so that she didn't have to look after her grandchildren like a typical granny.

'I won't take no for an answer,' said Mona, because she knew exactly what was going on in Shiela's mind. The friends knew of the situation in each other's homes, inside and out. Mona was willing to bet that she had not even told her husband about her problem and as usual, he was too busy to notice anything amiss. 'I'll pick you up and we'll take Meera along for the consult tomorrow but if there is anything serious, year-end closing or no closing, I'll see to it that your husband and sons come right away. Agreed?'

'Agreed,' said Shiela feebly.

***

While Mona and Meera waited outside, Dr Rosy took a detailed history, including that of medications for oral contraceptives and over-the-counter drugs like ginseng, could cause perimenopausal bleeding (PMB). After this, she carried out a thorough clinical examination and ruled out atrophic changes, vaginal, urinary and anal causes for bleeding—though they were infrequent, they had to be looked for nevertheless. What she did find was an irregularly enlarged uterus about the size of a five-month-old pregnancy!

When the other two friends were called in, the grave look on the face of the jovial doctor alarmed them.

'What is it, doctor?' asked Mona.

'Shiela has what we call perimenopausal bleeding (PMB), which could be due to anything ranging from fibroids (as I have found in her case), to polyps or endometrial hyperplasia—thickening of the inner lining of the uterus. This in turn could be due to hormonal imbalance or endometrial cancer (EC), so, an immediate evaluation is essential. We will have to do certain tests for confirmation of the diagnosis and look out for co-morbidities like diabetes and hypertension, but our immediate concern is severe anaemia due to excessive blood loss, for which she will need admission and blood transfusions.'

There was only so much friends could do, so Mona rang up Shiela's husband and told him about the whole situation. He immediately shut shop and came rushing to the hospital with both his sons. Nothing was more important that Shiela, her menfolk now realized. She was the pivot around which their household revolved and they had always taken her for granted, but not anymore. It took an illness as grave as this for them to realize how important she was to them. She had always underplayed her problems. This time, too, she had attributed her symptoms to impending menopause and ended up losing a lot of blood.

Anyway, she was admitted to the hospital and various tests were performed. Her haemoglobin was 4 gm per cent! It was a wonder that she was even able to stand with such low levels! Nothing definitive could be done about her bleeding till her haemoglobin reached at least 8 gm per cent. As her husband had diabetes, high blood pressure and mild angina, he was an unfit candidate for blood donation. Wonder upon wonders, not only her sons but their wives, Rama and Reena, willingly donated blood for her. Her illness had brought her family together. The fact that she was not an intimidating lady, but a very sick woman, brought out the best in the girls.

An ultrasound revealed a number of fibroids and a thickened inner lining, which was not a good sign. Dr Rosy was concerned that it could be endometrial cancer. Mona and Meera came to meet Shiela every day and prayed for her every night. A couple of days later, after four blood transfusions, with a bit of colour back in her cheeks, Shiela was wheeled into the operation theatre for a hysteroscopy dilatation and curettage (D&C) under general anaesthesia. This entailed inserting a telescope inside the uterine cavity after distending it with fluid and viewing the interior of the womb. Lying within was a huge polyp that could have contributed to the apparent thickness of the endometrium. Thankfully, it was one of the few benign lesions whose symptoms mimic cancer. A major load was lifted off their chests as the histopathology showed that the lesions were benign and not cancerous.

However, lying helplessly in the hospital, Shiela had time to think about her life and she realized that she needed to change her outlook. She made a conscious decision to be kinder going forward. So far, she had only appreciated result-oriented dedication because her efficient mind could not take people who were not at her level. This made her seem like a tyrant to her employees. She realized that instead of losing her patience with those less blessed, she should appreciate the hard work they put in to make up for their lack of efficiency. Perhaps the staff would learn to love her instead of fearing her. This reminded her of the poor girl, Mala, she had frightened out of her wits.

As for her household, she had run it with a commander-like rigidity like the formidable mother-in-law in the Rekha-starrer *Khubsoorat*. A person's true nature is revealed in times of crisis and despite the grudges they harboured against her, both Rama and Reena did not hesitate to donate blood for her. God bless them! From now on, she would encourage her daughters-in-law, appreciate their efforts and overlook their minor faults. The poor girls had left their parents' homes to live in hers and it was up to her to make the atmosphere more congenial.

A few days later, her irregularly enlarged uterus, studded with fibroids, was removed and Shiela got her wish—there would be no more periods. What she did not anticipate but got in abundance was love—from her family, especially her daughters-in-law, who looked after her as any daughter could have. As for her friends, Mona and Meera, they had literally saved her life!

Members of her staff too came to visit her every day, but the one her eyes sought never came. When she had almost given up hope, Mala entered her hospital room. The poor girl had been consumed with guilt because she thought that her curse had brought this catastrophe upon her beloved madam! How could she have forgotten that principal madam had given her a huge sum in advance when she had needed the money urgently after her brother's accident? Though she was always strict, it was madam's illness that had made her so sharp and snappy. Looking at Shiela lying on a hospital bed made her cry. 'Forgive me, madam, please forgive me,' she pleaded.

'For what?'

'I . . . I wished you were dead. That's why this has happened to you!' she blurted out.

'Do you really think that this happened because of you?' asked Shiela.

'Yes ma'am . . . er . . . no, madam,' stuttered the distraught girl.

'I will live on to keep scolding you!' said Shiela, smiling sweetly at her.

'Please do,' said Mala and they burst out laughing.

8

THE ELIXIR OF YOUTH
Hormone Replacement Therapy

Today was the corporate group's third session with Dr Rosy. From now on, it was decided that they would draw lots and decide what the majority wanted her to speak on. It turned out that this time, it was HRT, or hormone replacement therapy, they were most eager to learn about.

The previous session on sex in middle age had been a great hit and most of them had to put into practice what had been explained with such naughty humour. Intimacy had been resumed or strengthened in most households, to the pleasant surprise of the husbands. This contributed to the glow on their faces, the sensuality of their walk and their heightened laughter, which came with a general sense of well-being.

Today, they eagerly looked forward to learning about HRT, the purported 'elixir of youth', but were soon to be disappointed for, as Dr Rosy put it, 'Fools rush in where angels fear to tread.'

'What do you mean?' asked Mona.

'I'll tell you about that later but first, let me explain what HRT is all about. Oestrogen and progesterone are the two female sex hormones that are produced by the ovaries on maturation, which occurs at puberty. They convert a girl child into a woman, as seen by the development of breasts, the curvy feminine figure and the beginning of periods. During reproductive life, they are responsible for the woman's sexuality, conception, pregnancy and delivery and play an important part in the well-being of all her systems. After the reproductive period is over, hormones levels slowly decrease, leading to the end of periods, or menopause, as we call it.'

'But why is nature so unkind to women when men have all the advantages?' asked Rita.

'Unkind?' asked Dr Rosy, incredulous. 'God has been very kind to us. To the female of the species, He has entrusted *His* job of creation and nurturing. You must be familiar with the adage "As God could not be everywhere, He made mothers". But imagine doing that all your life and having no time at all for yourself. The postmenopausal years when, thankfully, worries about childbearing, child-rearing, abortion and contraception, menstruation and sanitary pads are over, is the bonus period He has rewarded you with to live life as you please!'

'I never thought of it that way,' said Rita.

'But how much can an old hag enjoy?' asked someone cheekily.

'How about starting by *not* becoming an old hag?' countered Dr Rosy.

'And how is that possible?'

'The medical profession thought of HRT as the elixir of eternal youth. They rationalized that if menopause was due to a decrease in levels of female hormones, replacement of these hormones would automatically reverse or delay the ageing process. Researchers thought that HRT would also reduce the ailments that accompany menopause, like a bunch of rowdy friends running rampant to negatively affect the heart, bone and bladder, besides the genital system. Pharmaceutical companies salivated at the thought of the huge market and the bigger profits to be obtained by development and sales of products that half the world population (the female half) would rush to buy. So they propagated with excitement the concept that HRT was the fountain of eternal youth, the panacea of all ills, and guess what? Female doctors were the first to try it!'

'Did you take it too?' asked Mona.

'Yes, I did,' Dr Rosy had the honesty to admit. 'But more for diseases I thought it would prevent. I have a very strong family history of blood pressure, diabetes and heart attacks. Little did I know then that all the propaganda that surrounded the advent of HRT was mere talk and the truth was exposed after the hype subsided. To my horror, my triglyceride levels increased! Triglycerides are fats that form plaques in arteries and make a person prone to heart disease and strokes—precisely what I was trying to avoid! Needless to say, I threw the offensive strip of tablets into the dustbin.'

'Then why was it promoted in such a big way?' asked Rita, puzzled.

'There is always great publicity about any new product that enters the market, but one must wait for further trials. Once, a long time ago, a drug called Thalidomide was introduced into the market in a big way to reduce morning sickness in pregnant patients. Sadly, it reduced not just the tendency to vomit but also the length of the limbs of the unborn foetus! After a number of babies were born with very short arms and legs to mothers who had taken Thalidomide, was the connection made and the drug withdrawn! What a disaster! Only after a new drug has been tried and tested for many years should one use it.'

'But by the time the trials end, it will be too late!' exclaimed Rita.

'Have patience. Women *my* age (and you are at least a decade younger to me) were happy that the drug came into the market at the exact time we needed it, but it did me more harm than good. Thankfully, you have the benefit of extensive trials that have been carried out since then and we have a clearer picture about its uses and side effects. Strict guidelines have emerged regarding the usage of HRT. I tell my patients that HRT is like a knife: useful if handled with care but can cut your hand if mishandled.'

'What was the trial about?'

'A study called HERS (the Heart and Estrogen/progestin Replacement Study) recruited 2,763 women (mean age: 66.7) for a period of 4.1 years between February 1993 and September 1994 at various trial centres and coordinated at the University of California, San Francisco.* It was done to see if HRT was of use in secondary prevention of coronary heart disease (CHD) in postmenopausal women, i.e., if it decreased further episodes of cardiac events and mortality rates in women with pre-existing heart problems. These women were divided into two groups: half were given HRT and the other half a placebo (dummy pill). To their utter surprise, those given HRT had more cardiac complications, that too within a period of a year, as compared to those who

*https://pubmed.ncbi.nlm.nih.gov/9683309/

received placebos. As if this was not enough, the chances of thrombo-embolism (blood clotting in veins which can cause heart problems, stroke and dementia) and gall bladder diseases increased, so the trial was stopped!'

As the group digested this unpalatable bit of information, Dr Rosy scared them further by stating that long-term use could sometimes lead to breast and endometrial cancer, and it did not prevent Alzheimer's or senile dementia, as originally thought.

'Then why have you prescribed it to me?' asked Pushpa, alarmed. She could live with hot flashes, but not cancers and heart disease.

'Calm down, Pushpa, let me explain. It isn't as if the medical fraternity has swung from one end of the pendulum to the other and ostracized HRT completely. HRT *is* being used judiciously and effectively for certain conditions, including yours. The trick is to give it in the lowest possible dose for the shortest possible period required, to bring about a cure. Rest assured, no harm will befall you.'

'Thank God!' said Pushpa relieved.

'HRT is definitely not an over-the-counter drug. It has to be used with caution under strict medical supervision only for a few select indications. These have been whittled down to the following:

- ♦ Moderate or severe menopausal symptoms
- ♦ Hot flashes and cold sweats
- ♦ Genitourinary: – like vaginal dryness and repeated urinary tract infection
- ♦ Premature menopause: natural/induced medically or surgically till the natural age of menopause
- ♦ Loss of bone mass

'It should be started as soon as symptoms appear, preferably before sixty years of age (even during the perimenopausal period) or within ten years of attaining menopause when the risk/benefit ratio is favourable. If initiated later, there is an increased risk of blood clotting in veins (though not with patches or gels), leading to coronary heart disease, stroke and dementia, as already stated.

♦ 'Though this is not an academic question, it is also important which drug is selected and for what. We have the option of giving oestrogen and progesterone together cyclically/continuously or either hormone singly, depending upon the situation. Your doctor will decide whether to give just oestrogen or combined oestrogen/progesterone pills, whether to give them continuously or cyclically depending upon whether you are in the perimenopausal period or have attained menopause and whether you or members of your family have other medical conditions. If a woman only has genitourinary symptoms, local application of oestrogen cream will suffice. Cyclical oestrogen progesterone (three weeks on, one week off) are given if debilitating vasomotor symptoms (hot flashes and cold sweats) appear in the perimenopausal period or after every three months if cycles are irregular. However, one must remember that **HRT is not a contraceptive**. Tibilone is another drug that can be used if there are side effects with HRT or if decreased libido is also an issue.

♦ Testosterone is being tried for decreased libido if the woman or her partner is distressed over her lack of sexual desire. It is marketed as Intrinsa patch abroad (and is not yet available in India), but can have side effects like masculinization and breast/endometrial cancer.

'I know, the talk is beginning to sound like a lecture for medical students, but all you have to remember is that your doctor will prescribe an appropriate HRT type, select its dose, route of administration and duration according to your need. That brings us to another important question: how long?

♦ Treatment should be individualized to maximize benefits and minimize risks.
♦ Usually, short-term HRT for five years (lifelong treatment was earlier considered) is recommended.
♦ Longer duration of therapy is considered for bone loss for the effect begins only after five years.

'Quite a didactic session, I think!' said Dr Rosy, smiling.

'Yes, but relevant nevertheless,' said Sheetal. 'Carry on, doctor, we asked for it; it *is* changing our ideas about HRT.'

'Okay, then, as we have seen, HRT is a double-edged sword that has to be used judiciously. So before starting it, your doctor will take a detailed history of pre-existing medical conditions like hypertension, diabetes, heart/liver/gall bladder disease, bleeding disorders that manifest as bruising easily, clotting in veins, stroke/depression/dementia, abnormal uterine bleeding and pre-existing cancers.

'They will then do a thorough general physical check-up, perform a breast and pelvic examination and send you for tests, which are mandatory before starting HRT and on a yearly follow-up. They include CBC (complete blood count), blood sugars, thyroid/liver/kidney function test and lipid profile. Besides these, ultrasound whole abdomen/TVS (transvaginal sonography), mammography and Pap smear will be done to diagnose pre-existing lumps in the breast, fibroids and precancerous conditions; to decide whether you are a fit candidate for HRT or not. Only after such a thorough evaluation will it be decided whether the benefits outweigh the risks. HRT is *not* given in women with undiagnosed abnormal genital bleeding, pre-existing breast/endometrial cancer, history of stroke, dementia, cardiac events, blood clotting in the veins, uncontrolled hypertension, liver disease and pregnancy.'

'Not that any of us *without* the above contraindications would want to use it,' said, one of the ladies present. They were getting more and more disillusioned with HRT. It was definitely not what they thought it would be.

'I understand your disappointment but to complete my talk, I have to tell you that once you are on HRT, you will be called after three months to see if you are tolerating it well or experiencing side effects that warrant a decrease in dosage or a change of medication. Some women experience spotting in the beginning of HRT, which may be normal, but they must report it to their doctor. Thereafter, you will be called yearly for a repeat examination and tests.'

'Quite a tedious, cumbersome procedure. Might as well take menopause in our stride and age gracefully,' spoke a small voice from the back.

'I know that I have scared you, but I have not come here to wave a magic wand like a fairy godmother, I only state the facts.'

'Is there no other way by which we can reverse or delay the ageing process?' asked another, reluctant to let go of hope.

'I was coming to that. There are non-hormonal preparations like antidepressants that help alleviate certain menopausal symptoms like hot flashes, but they have to be used with caution. Then there are the much-hyped bio-identical hormone preparations made from plant sources like soya that are being used in place of synthetic hormones, for it contains phyto-oestrogens—oestrogens from plant sources. It has been noticed that women in China, Japan and Korea appear more youthful than their counterparts in other countries; in fact, there is no word for hot flashes in Korean. Increased use of soya in their diet is thought to be responsible for it. You can increase the intake of soya and soya products like tofu and soya milk in your diet. However, drugs containing soya and other natural products for treating menopausal symptoms, like evening primrose oil, black cohosh, angelica, ginseng and St John's Wort, that are sold in health shops, should be considered with a pinch of salt. Some of them may reduce hot flashes, but generally, many complementary therapies aren't supported by scientific evidence. Yet others may cause serious side effects. For instance, ginseng can cause postmenopausal bleeding, which is definitely not acceptable!'

'We have ended up being more confused than ever,' lamented Malvika. 'So what do we do?'

'Simple,' said Dr Rosy. 'Those with symptoms like severe hot flashes, vaginal dryness, urge incontinence (inability to hold urine) or premature menopause may need HRT, though milder cases can be managed by lifestyle changes and the use of vaginal lubricants. As for those who have reached this milestone or are nearing it without any untoward symptoms, do what I told you in the first lecture.'

'We could do with a revision.'

'Well, menopause can be effectively managed by:

- ♦ Lifestyle changes – quit smoking, active or passive
- ♦ Avoid caffeine, alcohol and spicy foods
- ♦ Take a healthy, nutritious diet
- ♦ Increase intake of fruits, vegetables and soya
- ♦ Calcium and Vitamin D supplements
- ♦ Antioxidants and vitamins
- ♦ Maintain a healthy body weight
- ♦ Keep BP, sugar, cholesterol in check
- ♦ Dress lightly and in layers
- ♦ Regular exercise—at least thrice a week
- ♦ Yoga and meditation
- ♦ Do Kegel's exercises to prevent leakage of urine
- ♦ Remain sexually active—use water-based lubricants or hormonal cream if required
- ♦ Go for yearly preventive health check-ups
- ♦ Do whatever you are passionate about—religion, painting, writing or even gossiping with friends.

'Have you read the book *Ikigai*?'

Some women raised their hands.

'For the benefit of those who haven't, there is an island, Okinawa, in Japan that has the maximum number of centenarians living active healthy lives, which they attribute to their ikigai. This is a Japanese word which, when loosely translated means "the happiness of always being busy", a reason to jump out of bed every morning. All of us have an ikigai; some have found it and are supremely happy pursuing their passion (I am lucky to have two—my profession and my writing) while others have yet to find it. I urge those who are still floundering to find their ikigai, the one thing they like doing best of all. According to a Japanese proverb, "Only staying active will want you to live a hundred years", so stay interested in life and as sure as day follows night, life will retain its interest in you.

'I would like to end this session by asking you a question: what is that which you gain with age that you can never acquire in youth?'

'Wisdom.'

'Experience.'

'Yes, but what else?'

'Resignation, acceptance of things that you rebelled against earlier.'

'True,' said Dr Rosy. 'I even penned a poem to that effect some time back. Would you like to hear it?'

'Yes!' they all said.

'Well here it is:

I CRY
I cry for the lost ideals of youth,
That time and tide snatched from me.
Each compromise grabbed a handful
Till, my coffers were emptied.

The world was my oyster once,
In which, I hoped to find my pearl
Disillusioned, I gave up, leaving
A trail of broken shells behind.

I began by trying to conquer the world
And ended up being vanquished,
Enthusiasm, zeal, vigour and will.
I relinquished, one by one
I cry,
Over the tolerance that comes with age,
The knowledge that nothing will change,
The corruption, crime and injustice,
I've learnt to take in my stride.

The blood of youth gushes hot no longer,
My conscience has become immune,
I give in, give up in resignation and
Shut my eyes for an illusion of peace.'

'Beautiful.'

'Thanks, but these feelings were penned at a low point in my life; now, with my zest back, I realize that there is still so much we can do with a wealth of knowledge, wisdom and experience at our disposal, if we have the will. But this is not the answer to my question. Let me rephrase it: what is the best part of ageing?'

After waiting awhile for an answer that was not forthcoming, Dr Rosy answered the question herself. She said, 'Grandchildren! These little angels cannot inhabit your youth but make ageing worthwhile. There is no bond more precious; there is no one you will cherish more than a grandchild and there is no love more sublime than that of a grandchild's. If the price of that love be wrinkles on your face and grey in your hair, you will find yourself willing to pay it a hundred times over. Mark my words; you will remember them when you become grandmothers yourselves.'

9

HEARTACHE

Menopause and CAD
(Coronary Artery Disease)

'She died peacefully in her sleep,' they told the mourners sagaciously. How could they know for sure? For all you know, she might have struggled for breath in trying to call for help but not loud enough for anyone to hear, till finally, she was forced to give up and succumb. All this could have happened while *they* were sleeping peacefully. These were the thoughts that raced through Shiela's mind as she attended the funeral of one of her neighbours, whose family appeared smugly satisfied with the fact that their mother 'died peacefully in her sleep'. What they meant was that they found her dead in bed when *they* got up from a peaceful sleep. She gave herself a mental shake. Why let such morbid thoughts crowd her mind? The woman was dead and that was an irrefutable fact. How did it matter if she died after a struggle or in her sleep unless she could have been saved? And that, no one would ever know.

Barely a week later, Shiela and her friends Meera and Mona attended another funeral. This time, the sixty-eight-year-old neighbour had 'indigestion' that did not go away with Eno or Digene. Her solicitous son took her to a GP who did an ECG. On finding that it was normal, he gave her an injection of Pantoprazole for her acidity and sent her home, where she died soon after! Herein lay the importance of continual medical education. So busy was the GP in his practice that he did not have the time to attend seminars and workshops to update his knowledge. Medicine is a dynamic subject that needs frequent updating so that a doctor in active practice is conversant with newer modalities and medicines. This lapse cost the woman her life, for an ECG is normal initially in many cases of heart attacks. A timely reference to a cardiologist could have saved her life.

There was a spate of deaths in their colony that December, mostly postmenopausal women, which alarmed the three friends. An 'aunty' had excessive sweating and 'ghabrahat' (palpitations) and gave up the ghost before the doctor could be summoned. It was another case of a heart attack but surprisingly, without pain. Later, they learnt that people with diabetes have silent heart attacks that are often missed and this woman, they all knew, was on insulin.

Worried, the trio went to visit Dr Rosy, their one-point contact with the medical fraternity. She would know what was best for them. She told them that the female hormone oestrogen protects a woman's cardiovascular system for as long as she is menstruating. It keeps the inner layer of the blood vessels pliable, which allows them to expand to accommodate increased blood flow, which is required after exertion. As long as they are menstruating, fewer women suffer from CAD (coronary artery disease coronary arteries are blood vessels to the heart) than males of the same age. The protective effect of oestrogen is lost after menopause and women become as vulnerable as men to heart attacks and strokes. Physical inactivity, weight gain, high blood pressure, diabetes and high cholesterol levels are other contributory factors. Another difference between heart attacks in males and females is that women rarely present with typical symptoms of heart attack like pain on the left side of the chest radiating to the left arm. Instead, they have symptoms that are vague and atypical, as a result of which, the condition is diagnosed late, resulting in an increased mortality rate. In other words, *more women die after the first heart attack than men.*

A woman may have symptoms like:

- pain in unusual areas – lower jaw, neck, back, one or both arms
- excessive sweating
- breathlessness
- pain or discomfort in the upper abdominal area
- pressure, discomfort or squeezing sensation in the centre of the chest
- fatigue, nausea, light-headedness

'So what do we do?' asked Mona, alarmed, though she was the only one among the three who had not yet attained menopause.

'To decrease the risk of a heart attack,' said Dr Rosy, 'you need to do the following:

- Adopt a healthy lifestyle.
- Quit smoking, both active and passive.

- Eat a diet rich in fruits and vegetables, whole grains, low-fat dairy products, poultry, fish and nuts, while limiting red meat and sugary foods and beverages.
- Exercise at least thrice a week. According to the American Heart Association, women should aim for at least 150 minutes of physical activity a week, 30 minutes five times a week, to prevent heart disease. Those who need to lose weight should increase their exercise time to 300 minutes or more weekly, depending on individual needs. Walking, cycling, dancing or swimming—activities that use larger muscles at low resistance—are good aerobic exercises.
- Maintain a healthy body weight
- Go for yearly preventive health check-ups

'Those who have a family history of heart disease are particularly prone to it. They too can decrease the incidence by adopting the above measures,' said Dr Rosy.

'What about HRT? It contains oestrogens, doesn't it? Can we take them to decrease the incidence of heart attacks after menopause?' asked Meera.

'Initially, it was thought to be of help but after extensive trials, cardiologists have found that it does not reduce the risk and do not recommend its use for the prevention of heart disease.'

'So what do we do?' Mona asked, more urgently this time.

'Patience was never one of your virtues,' Dr Rosy said and smiled at Mona. 'I suggest that all three of you visit a heart doctor right away.' She reached for the intercom to refer them to a good cardiologist in her hospital.

So off they marched to the cardiology department, where they paid for a preventive cardiac health check-up and were asked to sit in the heart OPD. A nurse took their blood pressure, pulse, temperature, weight, measured their height, their waist and hip circumference and made them wait for their turn. Too nervous to make small talk, the three whiled away their time going through the heart health pamphlets on the centre table.

They learnt that taking into account their height and weight and using a certain formula, their body mass index (BMI) is measured. If it is more than 30, it isn't good, because obesity puts one at higher risk for health problems, especially heart disease. Also, the places where the fat accumulates—like your stomach or your hips—decide your fate.

Their waist and hip circumferences were taken to calculate the waist-hip ratio precisely for this reason. Broadly speaking, those with 'apple-shaped' bodies (more weight around the waist) faced more health risks than those with 'pear-shaped' bodies (more weight around the hips). People with abdominal obesity, i.e., a waist-hip ratio above 0.90 for males and above 0.85 for females, are at a higher risk for heart disease. This was news to the three women, who discussed it at length. They also learnt that if, besides being overweight, they had one more additional risk factor, the chances of getting CAD increased manifold. These risk factors were:

- ♦ Diabetes
- ♦ Blood pressure
- ♦ Smoking
- ♦ Family history of CAD
- ♦ Deranged lipid profile—high bad cholesterol LDL, low good cholesterol HDL and high triglycerides

that cause the development of plaque in the inner lining of arteries, which narrows and stiffens them. This does not allow them to expand when more blood is required after exertion, stress etc. If such a thing happens in the coronary arteries, it leads to angina (myocardial ischaemia)—pain in the chest on exertion—heart attacks (myocardial infarction) during which a part of the heart tissue dies, due to complete blockage of the blood vessel with plaques or clots. If the narrowing/blockage of blood vessels occur in the brain, it leads to stroke and paralysis.

High blood pressure and diabetes usually have no symptoms in the initial stages, hence the importance of regular preventive health check-ups.

The cardiologist, Dr Puneet Verma, was a handsome man, lean and fit, with a pleasant smile and an easy manner. It does put one off to have an overweight doctor telling you to lose weight or one who smokes and drinks ordering you not to do so, though a board in her GP's office did bring a smile to Meera's lips. It read:

'DO AS I SAY, NOT AS I DO'

After all, doctors too are human.

He examined them thoroughly and gave them basic instructions that Dr Rosy and the patient information booklets had already given them. The third time around, the instructions were fixed permanently in their minds. The moot point was, would they follow them?

Meera's blood pressure was borderline high, while Shiela's was positively high. The doctor wrote down a list of blood tests that would be done the next day, for the lipid and thyroid profile and fasting blood sugar tests had to be done on an empty stomach. Other tests included compete blood count (CBC), liver function test (LFT), kidney function test (KFT) and urine routine examination.

Meanwhile, all three had an ECG done, which was normal. This was followed by a stress echo, wherein one by one, they were wired up and connected to a screen that showed continuous ECG readings as they walked on a treadmill with increasing speed till their heart rates reached a certain level. After this, they were made to bare their chests while the handsome doctor did an ultrasound examination of the heart. The beautiful Mona with her magnificent breasts could not tell whether her palpitation was due to the handsome doctor's closeness or her running on the treadmill (the presence of a female nurse notwithstanding)!

Meera was too scared to think such naughty thoughts; in fact, she was embarrassed by her floppy breasts that fell, one on each side, on opening her hospital gown, for they had been made to remove their bras. As for Shiela, she was terrified, for she had not been able to run on the treadmill due to her obesity and had to be given an injection to increase her heart rate to the desired levels. To her dismay, the doctor found a fault in her echo and said that she needed further evaluation, including an angiography. If there was a blockage, she might need a stent.

Back in Mona's car, Shiela was on the verge of tears. The other two consoled her by saying that it was good they had decided to visit the doctor *before* something untoward happened and it was possible to take preventive measures before severe damage occurred.

They returned a few days later with their test reports. Mona was perfectly fit, while Meera was a borderline case.

She had borderline obesity, and her blood pressure, sugars and lipids and TSH levels were borderline high. She was advised to visit a dietician for diet modifications, given an exercise regimen and medicine for hypothyroidism, which was to be taken on an empty stomach each morning. Meera thanked her stars that these problems were caught before they got out of hand and was determined to do whatever it took to reduce her weight and regain her health.

As for Shiela, she was in a fix. Despite having a large, loving joint family, she had no one who would stay with her in the hospital in case she needed a stent or two. She was not scared of the procedure as such because there were many she knew who were doing well after the procedure. What worried her was the lack of help during those crucial days in the hospital and post-operative care at home. It so happened that her husband had hurt his leg and needed a walker these days. Though he still hobbled to his accountancy firm, which he ran with his two sons (all three being chartered accountants), he would be of no use as a nursemaid. Her elder son was travelling abroad with his wife and therefore the management of the office was on the shoulders of her younger son and the management of the house on his wife's.

In desperation, she rang up a cousin who was a cardiologist in the US and told him about her predicament. He tried to pacify her by saying that the stress echo could give false positive reports sometimes.

'But what if I do need a stent? I have no one to look after me!' she wailed and, after a moment's hesitation, she voiced another secret fear. She had heard rumours of mercenary doctors who, after scaring a patient out of her wits during the course of an angiography, inserted unnecessary stents in normal arteries, inserting along with it a lifetime of fear in patients who were *not* heart patients.

'This doctor is highly recommended, and I do not think he will do such a thing but . . .' her voice trailed off.

'You can always ask for a DVD of the procedure . . .' he began, but then an idea struck him. 'Why don't you go for a thallium stress test?'

'What's that?' she asked.

'It is an imaging study that measures your blood flow during rest and after exercise that too, without any form of intervention.'

'What do you mean?'

'Though the test gives a clear picture of the blood flow to your heart, it is not invasive, unlike angioplasty (where a catheter is already in place in your vein and you have to take an instant decision), you can postpone the stenting, if required, to a convenient date. It will solve all your problems,' he said excitedly.

So she duly went for a thallium stress test and it was found, much to her relief, that her angina was of a mild variety. It could be managed by medication and lifestyle changes, to which she happily agreed. That she was overweight and had hyperlipidemia, hypertension and diabetes were matters of concern which needed lifestyle modifications, yet more medicines and strict follow-ups, but so grateful was she to the Almighty for sparing her an intervention that she was more than willing to do anything to protect her heart.

These three friends highlighted the fact that one in three females in the older age group has some form of cardiovascular disease. If screening test results are less than ideal, do not get stressed. Be thankful that you have been warned in time to make the right changes. However, if active preventive measures are not taken even during this window period, it bodes ill because there is an overall increase in heart attacks among women, usually ten years after menopause. In fact, it is the leading cause of death in women the world over.

Friendly advice: preventive cardiac health check-ups are a must. If the predisposing factors are corrected, if the disease is caught early and managed appropriately you have a long and fruitful life ahead of you.

10

LIVING IN THE CLOUDS

Shiela was busy preparing for an important meeting with the trustees of her primary school. A lot depended on this. As a principal, she had much on her hands but, till now, the responsibilities had only enhanced her efficiency. Though a formidable person to reckon with (at least in her official avatar), she realized to her dismay that she was slipping. She had begun to forget names and her mind would become blank in the middle of a conversation. While the person waited patiently for her to continue, she could not remember what she wanted to say, however hard she tried. This made her irritable and she would snap at her staff for no reason. Perhaps, she had taken too much on herself and wondered if the chronic fatigue was taking its toll. Anxieties kept her up at nights, and her mind was plagued with what would become of her if her condition persisted. The insomnia led to further lack of concentration and temporary loss of memory which worsened the situation.

She could have borne any physical disability, but the failing of mental faculties was unbearable. 'Was this the beginning of the end? Was it Alzheimer, but at this age? I am only fifty-four years old!,' she deliberated about the cause frantically. She did have her uterus removed for excessive menstrual bleeding about eighteen months back, but surely there was no connection between her reproductive system and her brain.

She had an efficient secretary, Supriya, and of late Shiela had begun to depend on her more and more. Supriya would take detailed notes so that Shiela could refer to them in case she forgot. For the presentation to the trustees too, Supriya had thoughtfully written the names of the trustees in the garb of a 'meeting with Misters so and so' on the top and listed the agenda in bullet points. Just then Shiela asked her to get a file from the cabinet.

'Which file?'

'That one?'

Supriya was smart and she knew that the trustees would want to go over the finances before investing more money in the school. Of her own accord, she brought the income tax file that contained details of their income and the expenditure incurred.

Shiela gave Supriya a grateful look. 'I must remember to give her a raise,' thought Shiela, though, she knew this was but a short-term solution.

She decided to go for a holiday by the sea after this blessed meeting was over. Maybe, watching the endless waves chase each other to the shore would soothe her troubled mind; the stunning sunsets, the silvery moonbeams on rippling water, would clear the fog from her brain. Reading a book on a hammock under swaying palms would distract her and the cool sea breeze would brace her spirits. A long walk bare-feet in the wet sand would induce sleep and she would come back rejuvenated.

After the meeting was over, she did take a break and went for a vacation. She felt better and there was less clutter in her brain, but the mist in mind continued to cloud her thinking. She was prone to headaches and mental fatigue that led to a lack of concentration and memory lapses. She would lose her keys, forget why she entered a room or why she opened the fridge. It embarrassed her no end to forget the names of people she knew.

Matters came to a head when she was walking in the park with her friends Mona and Meera.

'I chucked her out,' she stated as if they both knew exactly whom she was talking about.

'Who?' asked Meera. For the life of her Shiela could not remember the name.

'That-that girl . . . she was caught stealing.'

'Who was caught stealing?' asked Mona.

At this, Shiela sat down with a thump on a park bench and broke down.

'I think I am losing my mind. I forget names and things and I cannot concentrate. My brain fogs over and I cannot think straight. This has affected my efficiency and my sleep. I just don't know what to do,' she said between sobs.

Mona and Meera were shocked. They had never seen the strong, self-sufficient Shiela so out of control.

'There, there, don't cry,' said Meera hugging her, while Mona held her hand and stroked it gently.

After the initial outburst subsided, Shiela lamented, 'I am sure I have Alzheimer. I cannot bear the thought of forgetting you both too.'

'You'd better not,' threatened Mona, playfully.

'I used to laugh at a joke about an old man who would call his wife by endearments like "Darling", "Honey", "Luv" and people would think that he loved her so much even at that age till he revealed that he had forgotten her name years ago. God forbid that I forget *your* names.'

'I, for one, wouldn't mind being called by such names,' smiled Meera.

'Things can't be that bad,' said Mona. 'You remembered the joke well enough. *I* remember what Dr Rosy had told me once. "If you remember that you don't remember, you don't have Alzheimer." Let's go to her'

'For you Mona, Dr Rosy is the one go-to person for any medical problems. She is a gynaecologist, *yaar*. What connection could the brain possible have with the vagina?' asked Meera with an exasperated smile, but Mona was adamant.

'What's the harm in going to her? Even if it is a neurologist or a psychologist that we need, she can guide us to the best there is.' And that was that.

The next day all three found themselves in Dr Rosy's clinic, while Shiela poured her woes into sympathetic ears.

'We know that this is not a gynaecological problem,' said Meera apologetically, 'but your die-hard fan Mona insisted on bringing us to you.'

To their surprise Dr Rosy said, 'And she was right.'

'What do you mean?' asked Shiela perplexed.

'Some women suffer from "brain fog" around menopause.'

'But you removed my uterus one and half years ago.'

'Yes, but not your ovaries. In your case, a hysterectomy led to the cessation of periods, not menopause. The uterus is but an end organ that responds to ovarian hormones by menstruating or nurturing pregnancies. It is when the ovaries stop functioning that a woman attains menopause. In your case, the ovaries continued to produce female sex hormones oestrogen and progesterone till now. Besides the female genital tract, almost all the other systems in a female's body need females sex hormones for optimal functioning. These, start getting affected once the ovaries pack up.'

'What other systems get affected?' asked Shiela.

'Almost every organ, right from the heart, skin, bladder, bone, breast and brain get affected.'

'Brain!' exclaimed Shiela and Mona in unison while Mona gave them I-told-you-so look.

'As oestrogen level decrease, you can have mild memory loss and a general fogginess of the brain. You could exist in a state of dysphoria—feeling very unhappy, uneasy, or dissatisfied. All this is loosely called "brain fog" or mental fatigue. It is also characterised by cognitive issues like:

♦ memory lapse
♦ lack of mental clarity
♦ poor concentration'

'Exactly what I have been experiencing,' said Shiela, nodding her head. 'But, the moot point is that can it be cured or it is a downhill struggle from now on?'

'Have patience. I will come to that.'

'Please understand doctor, the very quality of my life is at stake.'

'It does not have to be a permanent fixture in your life but first tell me, do you have sleep disturbances?'

'Yes.'

'Hot flashes and night sweats?'

'At times.'

'And they did not bother you?'

'I thought that they were a natural part of aging.'

'Though the insomnia could be due to causes other than oestrogen deficiency, hot flashes are because of this. These two combined together are enough to decrease one's efficiency and HRT (hormone replacement therapy) will definitely help. You'll feel better, get proper sleep, your focus and memory will return

Even in as Shiela nodded in eager consent, Mona put a spoke in her wheel.

'But HRT has many harmful side-effects. You said so yourself in the class you took in my office some time back.'

Shiela looked from one to the other in bewilderment.

'Given for a short term (less than five years) at the right time, for specific conditions, under strict medical supervision it works wonders, but if one is wary of taking HRT, we could try other things.'

'Like what?' asked Shiela.

'Before I go into all that, let me tell you that thyroid conditions can also give rise to the above symptoms. Both hypothyroidism (an underactive thyroid gland) and hyperthyroidism (an overactive thyroid gland) can lead to memory loss and other cognitive problems. Besides, routine tests like haemoglobin (remember anaemia was the cause of your irritability when you had excessive menstrual blood loss), we will also do a complete thyroid profile. In that case, all you need is a tablet a day to clear the fog in the brain.'

'Really, I wish . . .' began Shiela but Mona steered the conversation back to brain fog.

'What other measures will cure or, for that matter, prevent brain fog? Perhaps Meera and I too could benefit by taking such measures.'

'Definitely,' said Dr Rosy, 'But, there is no magic formula. Lifestyle modifications are all that you need. Ensure that you rest enough, sleep well in a well-ventilated room in cotton night wear on cotton sheets, eat a balanced and nutritious diet with plenty of green leafy vegetables, get proper exercise (thirty mins for at least five time a day), practice relaxation techniques like yoga and meditation and, maintain an optimal weight. It is very important to keep you brain active to prevent fogging and the other mental issue associated with aging. A brain workout includes:

- ♦ Doing crossword puzzles and Sudoku.
- ♦ Playing word games, online brain games and quizzes.
- ♦ Reading books, newspapers, and magazines.
- ♦ Learning something new, like a musical instrument or a new language.
- ♦ Spend time talking and socializing with family or friends.'

'That I will definitely do,' said Shiela fervently.

'So will we,' said the other two.

Six months later, Shiela lost twelve kgs—partly due to her diet and exercise regimen and partly due to the medication for hypothyroidism. She felt so much lighter and good about herself. Best of all, it improved her mental status too. The atmosphere at school was congenial now that they had a calmer and kinder principal. She slept well, was less forgetful, less irritable and almost back to being her original efficient self. The three friends had taken

Dr Rosy's advice seriously. Soon, they were busy learning new things in life—while Mona was taking French lessons, Meera and Shiela were learning to play the sitar and tabla from a nearby music school—and they were enjoying themselves thoroughly.

Friendly advice: Do not panic when you suffer from minor memory losses with advancing age. It is part of aging process that can be reversed, and you are not necessarily heading towards dementia. Seek medical advice at the earliest.

11

BROKEN BONES

Osteoporosis

Maya Devi, or Mataji, as she was called, was a sprightly lady eighty years of age. Her frailty belied her inner strength, for she was active and quite capable of looking after herself. She would get up at 5 a.m., bathe *and* wash her own clothes. After peeling and eating the almonds she had soaked overnight, she would dress in a crisp white cotton sari, plait her sparse white hair and wind her ancient wristwatch. It had been given to her by her husband shortly before he died, forty years ago, and she would not exchange it for any of the fancy watches her son Manohar gave her. All spruced up and ready, she wore her glasses and walked to the local mandir, which was over half a kilometre away. On her return, she would eat a light breakfast of *upma* or *poha* or porridge that Meera, her daughter-in-law, kept ready for her. Her diet was frugal, healthful and eaten at appropriate intervals. A bowl of fresh fruit at 11 a.m., lunch of khichdi or sabzi roti at 1 p.m., tea with a biscuit at 5 p.m., to the mandir again in the evening, followed by a light dinner at 8 p.m. She would then retire to her room with a glass of milk and go off to sleep by 9 p.m. It was this clockwork routine and strictness of protocol that Meera had found difficult in her early years as a daughter-in-law, but now wished she could do the same because she could see that it had contributed greatly to the health, agility and longevity of the old woman. Meera understood her mother-in-law better and liked her more with the passage of years for now she, too, had matured. Mataji was no trouble at all for she did not throw her weight around—not that she had much weight to throw around. Instead, she helped with the tedious work of plucking fenugreek leaves, cutting vegetables, peeling fruit, cleaning the tiny mandir they kept at home and lighting *kapoor* (camphor), which kept mosquitoes at bay without chemicals. She did not grudge Meera the time she spent walking and talking with her friends Shiela and Mona in the evening. In fact, they too loved Mataji, especially the *besan ke laddoos* full of dry fruits she made for them using desi ghee every Diwali.

Manohar sat with his mother for half an hour every evening when he returned from office, which satisfied her as a mother as well. At times, to relive his childhood, Manohar would ask his mother to prepare foods that she specialized in, like *zarda*—sweet saffron basmati rice with almonds— and instead of being jealous, Meera gladly handed the kitchen to her. She was also grateful to Mataji for taking charge of her grandchildren when her daughters visited, so that she could gossip with them undisturbed. Mataji's great-grandchildren loved her. She would open her secret box and hand out goodies, after which, with the younger ones settled on her lap, she told them stories from the Ramayana and the Mahabharata; later, she gave ten-rupee coins to those who answered her questions on these epics correctly. With her silver hair, cataract-greyed eyes, her crumpled, parchment-like skin over her fine bone structure, her ready smile and her rimless glasses, she looked like a benevolent character from one of these epics herself.

'It is a blessing to have such an elder in the house,' thought Meera with a sigh of contentment as she prepared her breakfast. But it seemed like she'd thought too soon, for the very next moment, she was startled by the urgent ringing of the doorbell. She rushed to find out whose finger was stuck to the doorbell, only to see the excited ten-year-old child of her neighbours.

'Aunty, aunty, I saw Mataji stumble on a stone and fall; she is not able to get up.'

'Oh no! Take me to her at once,' said Meera, rushing out, though she had the presence of mind to turn the gas off and lock the door before leaving.

By the time the two reached the spot, a crowd had gathered. A kindly gentleman had picked up the frail old lady and put her down on a bench in the park, while another held a glass of water to her lips. Both her forearms were swollen and bruised and appeared deformed; she was in pain and moaned softly. With the help of her neighbours, Meera got her home and with her husband, she took her to the orthopaedic specialist. X-rays revealed that she had fractured both her forearms while trying to stop her fall with her outstretched hands. It was called a Colles fracture and usually occurred in elderly postmenopausal women.

Maya Devi was a fracture waiting to happen; given her age, frailty and calcium-depleted bones, they broke like twigs upon the minimal trauma that healthy bones could have easily withstood. As it is, the risk of falls increases with age due to poor vision and balance issues. It is as if the cement had crumbled out of a building's pillars, and a flimsy hollow structure stood in its place, which gave way to the slightest of force.

'This is the third fragility fracture I have come across in this week,' said Dr Amar Jain, the orthopaedic specialist, with some degree of annoyance. He was unhappy about the fact that people did not take precautionary measures to avoid such preventable accidents. Seeing his confused patient, he explained, 'After menopause, bones lose calcium rapidly and become fragile, leading to a condition called osteoporosis. It is a silent process that becomes apparent when bones break after minor injuries.'

Then putting a hand gently on Mataji's shoulder, he said, 'We will reduce the fractures under anaesthesia and put both your arms in a cast, but first, let me relieve you of your pain.'

Tears streamed from Maya Devi's eyes, not only because of the pain, but because of the fact that she would be dependent on others for her day-to-day living. Her son took off her specs and lovingly wiped her eyes with his handkerchief.

'Will she be alright?' he asked anxiously.

'It will take time but I am hopeful that she will recover.'

The doctor was deliberately vague about the time for he did not want to demoralize them by saying that, given the state of her bones, it could take up to a year. He ordered a few urgent tests that were required before anaesthesia, to which he added testing of calcium and Vitamin D levels. He would test her bone density by DEXA (Dual Energy X-ray Absorptiometry) later, when she came for a follow-up visit. As expected, her calcium and Vitamin D levels were very low and the DEXA reports way too bad. Thankfully, she did not have any other co-morbidities like blood pressure, diabetes, heart disease or thyroid disease. On discharge, she would be prescribed high doses of calcium tablets and Vitamin D sachets, besides painkillers.

While her mother-in-law lay in the recovery room, Meera decided, and rightly so, that she needed a personal consult with the bone specialist. Though Dr Amar Jain appeared intimidating, he had been strongly recommended for his expertise and experience and advice was what Meera now needed. She did not want to end up in the situation Mataji found herself in, which, he said was preventable. Her husband agreed wholeheartedly and let her go as Mataji was still deeply sedated; he was by her side and the nurse was but a ring of the bell away.

So, Meera found herself facing the solemn Dr Jain for the second time in the day.

'What can I do to avoid getting into the situation Mataji has landed herself in?' she asked.

'I like it when people come asking for prevention, instead of coming when they need treatment,' he said, though not a trace of a smile appeared on his grim face.

Meera waited for him to continue.

'Bone is a dynamic tissue which undergoes continuous remodelling with the formation of new bone and absorption of old bone. A mismatch of this process forms the basis of osteoporosis, a condition in which there is a decrease in the density of bone mass.

'Osteoporosis is asymptomatic, as in, you have it till a fracture occurs. Diagnosis of the condition during the asymptomatic period, and timely management, prevents fragility fractures, with their associated morbidity and mortality.'

'Mortality?'

'Yes, if the hip bone or the pelvic bones fracture, the patient, especially an elderly one, is bedridden or confined to a wheelchair for the rest of their life, or at least for a very long time. The lack of mobility leads to a decrease in lung function (unless regular breathing exercises are performed with the help of a physiotherapist), collection of fluid in the lungs and death in the span of year or two.'

'That is scary; so what can I do?' she asked.

'It is a good idea to take milk, calcium and Vitamin D3 supplements from the age of thirty-five onwards. If you haven't done so yet, please start now and tell your friends and relatives around this age also to do so, for once osteoporosis develops, more vigorous treatment is required. It is commoner in females, especially in the perimenopausal age group, as the protective effect of oestrogen begins to decrease.'

'Protective effect of oestrogen?' asked Meera.

'Yes, oestrogens help retain calcium in the bone. After menopause, calcium is depleted rapidly, leading to decreased bone strength and increase in bone fragility, with a susceptibility to fractures usually involving the wrist, spine, hip, pelvis, ribs and upper arm.'

'How will I know if I just need supplements, or I have already developed osteoporosis?'

'In a previously healthy woman, it takes at least five years after menopause for osteoporosis to set in. However, if you have osteopenia (low bone mass), which is the middle stage, we can diagnose it by doing a bone densitometry (DEXA is the best method), get your calcium and Vitamin D levels tested, and treat you accordingly.'

'I see.'

'Another thing,' he added, smiling for the first time since Meera met him, 'frail women are more likely to get fractures than those who are on the heavier side.'

He did have a nice smile, thought Meera—someone should tell him to smile more often.

'That means I am protected,' said Meera, laughing self-consciously, for she was a little on the heavier side.

'Maybe,' he smiled again, 'but you will be more prone to diabetes, thyroid disease, high blood pressure and heart problems, so there is no escaping the process of ageing.'

'True,' she said.

'Another thing: thyroid disease and diabetes predispose a person to secondary osteoporosis.'

'Really?' she asked, subdued, for she had mild hypothyroidism and was on medication for the same.

'Try to keep your weight under control and do some sort of exercise every day.'

'I go for a walk every evening with my friends.'

'Good. Add weight-bearing exercises twice a week at least to your schedule. What about your diet?'

'I think it is fairly well-balanced but if could you tell me which food contains calcium, it would be of great help.'

'The intake of calcium should be 600 mg in adults and 800 mg in postmenopausal women, and this includes dietary intake. Roughly one glass of cow milk has 300 gm of calcium and one *katori* (bowl) cow milk curd has 149 mg calcium, while one glass of buffalo milk has 525 gm of calcium and one katori curds from buffalo milk has 300 mg calcium. Though dairy products have the maximum amount of calcium, other calcium-rich foods are green leafy vegetables, legumes, figs etc.'

'Doctor, people say that calcium intake leads to kidney stones and heart issues.'

'Not in the amount we advise you to take.'

'Thank you, Doc, for clearing my misconception. Can we get Vitamin D from natural sources?'

'God has been bountiful in giving us so much sunlight, but we avoid it. We stay indoors most of the time, slather ourselves with sunscreen lotion when we go out and hardly allow the golden rays to work their magic,' he said.

Meera remembered the time she had come as a newlywed to this colony. Old ladies sitting on string charpoys in the sun, knitting, gossiping, plucking fenugreek leaves; naked grandchildren glistening by their sides after a thorough massage with mustard oil, was a common sight. Nowadays, there was not a soul outdoors. All sat huddled inside with ACs or heaters on, according to the season.

'For how long should we sit the sun?' she asked.

'Expose 20 per cent of your body surface area (face, neck and both arms and forearms) to sunlight without sunscreen for at least 30 minutes between 10 a.m. and 3 p.m. After menopause, it is advisable to take Vitamin D supplementation in addition to sunlight exposure to reduce the incidence of fractures.'

'So Mataji's fracture could have been prevented,' said Meera, thoughtfully. 'If we only knew what I know now.'

'Elderly women tend to lose height too.'

'How is that possible?'

'Sometimes, there is compression fracture of the vertebra (the spinal column) with or without pain. If you recollect the elderly women of *your* childhood, you must remember at least one with a hunched back.'

'Yes, my *bhabhi* mother had a pronounced hunchback.'

'Thankfully, we do not see such severe cases of osteoporosis these days,' he said.

'Yes.'

'So, tell me, what will you do for your bone health from today onwards?'

'I will increase the calcium in my diet, start taking calcium tablets, sit in the sun and take Vitamin D supplements after getting my blood tested for Vitamin D deficiency. As for exercise, I am already taking a brisk walk for an hour daily. I will add some weight-training exercises. I will also make sure that my friends and neighbours who are above thirty-five years of age also follow your advice.'

'You have summed it up beautifully, though I will add a few more words of caution. Decrease your caffeine intake to three cups a day and salt to less than one teaspoon a day. Also, no smoking and no alcohol, and do not overload the knee joint by squatting or frequent climbing down the stairs,' said the doctor.

'But I was told that squatting keeps the knee joint flexible and climbing up and down the stairs is good for health.'

'Climbing up the stairs puts a strain on the heart and climbing down strains the knee joint, while squatting strains the ligaments of the knee joint. If these are already strained due to age, obesity etc., the added pressure will make them more vulnerable. For a knee joint replacement surgery to be successful, it is important that the ligaments are healthy. This is because we replace the worn-out bone and need normal ligaments to keep the joint intact.'

'Scary. One last question, doctor. When should we get a DEXA done?' asked Meera.

'It should be done in all older women at five years after menopause and in women with fragility fractures like your mother-in-law. It is also done in postmenopausal women within five years of menopause if they have risk factors like frailty, low calcium and Vitamin D levels, diabetes, thyroid dysfunction or those who have radiological evidence of osteopenia (low bone mass). Women with osteoporosis need a baseline DEXA before initiating treatment and for monitoring the treatment when it is repeated between one and five years later, depending upon individual risk factors.'

'What about camps where, among other things, they test the bone density of your heel?'

'Heel bone densitometry is a rough screening method for the mass population, but the bone density of the hip and spine regions give an accurate picture.'

'Thank you, doctor, for vastly increasing my knowledge,' said Meera gratefully.

'About your mother-in-law, a lady who once had a fragility fracture is prone to having it again, so make your house hazard-free to minimize chances of a fall. Thankfully, it was the wrists this time, but if she breaks her hip bone or back, you all have had it. Her calcium tablets will continue lifelong while she takes D sachets weekly for at least ten weeks. After that, I will reassess and let you know. In any case, after the deficiency has been corrected, the dose will be reduced to once a month in the summers and twice a month in the winters for maintenance. Do not self-medicate. People tend to think that more is better, but not with Vitamin D. Excess amounts can lead to toxicity.'

'Got it.'

'After Mataji's plaster is removed, she will need physiotherapy. Meanwhile, give her emotional support and help her regain her self-confidence so that she becomes independent once again.'

'I have read an article in which the doctor mentioned the use of HRT in bone loss. Can we give it to Mataji?'

'Not at this age; definitely not to women who are more than ten years postmenopausal.'

'Mataji stopped having her periods forty years ago, soon after her husband died.'

'Moreover, to be of use in osteoporosis, HRT should be started in the perimenopausal period and taken for at least five years, that too after calculating the risk-benefit ratio. Also, as in her case, once osteoarthritis sets in, HRT offers no protection. In such cases, osteoarthritis should be treated on its own merits—early osteoarthritis can be addressed by lifestyle modification, medication and physiotherapy, while advanced osteoarthritis needs surgical intervention such as total knee replacement.'

'Thank you, doctor, thank you very much,' said Meera.

With both hands in plaster, Mataji's life was a disaster, at least initially. In place of crisp cotton saris, she was clad in a maxi with cut sleeves and with large armholes, night and day. Their maid Laxmi was paid to stay for the extra time she devoted to bathing Mataji, combing her hair and washing her clothes. Meera prepared nutritious broths and fed her lovingly as if she was her own mother. Not a frown creased her homely face, which now appeared to Mataji as that of an angel; she blessed Meera from the bottom of her heart. Her son put chants and bhajans on her ancient CD player for her to listen to and read the Bhagwad Gita aloud to her for half an hour every evening. Her granddaughters and great-grandchildren visited her often. The children enjoyed having their way with her. They drew funny faces on her plaster and hugged and kissed her. Besides the little titbits they brought, Meera's friends Shiela and Mona gave Mataji the most precious gift of all—their time. They took to sitting by her instead of on the bench in the park every evening after their walk. Her mandir mates, old women like herself, too came to meet her as often as they could. Never by word or by deed did anyone make her feel that she was a burden to the family. Mataji could only thank the heavens for showing her how much she was loved and wanted. She had been a giver all her life and for the first time, experienced the joy of receiving.

After a few weeks, Mataji's plaster was removed; the fractures healed remarkably well for her age. Life was back to normal, with some modifications. Besides the calcium and Vitamin D she took as advised, her visits to the mandir were reduced to once a day, that too by car with her son. As for her evening walk, instead of the pebble-strewn road to the temple, Meera accompanied her to the park gate, where they separated, each walking with her own set of friends at different paces on the smooth walking track around a verdant lawn. All was well with their world again. As for Meera, after the session with Dr Jain, she saw to it that there wasn't single lady above thirty-five years in the park who was not taking her daily dose of calcium tablets!

Bone Health In Postmenopausal Period

- Calcium in the diet, and calcium tablets
- Exposure to sun and Vitamin D supplements after testing
- Brisk walk daily
- Weight training exercises twice a week
- Minimise the use of stairs and squatting
- Bone densitometry test to be done for early diagnosis of osteoporosis

12

IT HUNG OUT ALL THERE
Prolapsed Uterus

It was while Laxmi, the maid, attended to Mataji during her convalescence after bilateral wrist fractures that she discovered Mataji's most well-kept secret. It embarrassed Mataji to be bathed by someone else but there was no alternative. As Laxmi was soaping her down below, she saw something unusual—a pinkish mass protruding from her vagina.

'*Yeh kya* (What's this), Mataji?' she asked, trying to hide her horror as best as she could.

'*Kuch nahi* (Nothing),' said Mataji mortified at being thus exposed.

'*Kuch toh hai. Iske saath aap chal kaise paati hai* (It *is* something. How can you even walk with this)?'

'I just push it in and wear a tight panty when I have to walk. It has been there for years and I have got used to living with it.'

It is amazing what a human can get used to, thought Laxmi.

'Don't tell Meera anything about it,' pleaded Mataji, but Laxmi could keep quiet only for so long.

She waited till Mataji's plaster was cut and she was able to fend for herself like before that she blurted everything out to her mistress. As she had dreaded all along, her daughter-in-law insisted on taking Mataji to a gynaecologist. The old lady looked reproachfully at Laxmi, who lowered her eyes.

'Child, I have lived with it for so many years, let's wait for a few more months. The plaster has just been removed; it will take some more time for the fracture to heal completely, and then we can go,' said Mataji.

Meera agreed but soon another complication cropped up. During the time her wrists were in plaster, Mataji was unable to push the 'thing' inside and it had chafed against her underwear leading to what was called a 'decubitus ulcer'. This bled off and on and the poor lady had to be taken to Dr Rosy sooner than she liked.

On examination Dr Rosy saw that Mataji had third-degree utero-vaginal prolapse—the vagina lay outside her body like a bag turned inside-out with the uterus in it. To have lived with this for so long! Though not life threatening, it definitely affected the quality of life. At that time there was a soreness at the tip of the protrusion that bled on touch.

'She needs a surgery,' said Dr Rosy, 'but we will wait for a month or so. Firstly, to allow the decubitus ulcer to heal. I will prescribe antibiotics and local antiseptic lotion to hasten the process.   I will also give her oestrogen cream for vaginal application twice a day so that the vaginal skin that has become tough and leathery due to years of exposure and oestrogen depletion with become soft and supple. This will make it easier to separate the various layers during surgery.'

That decided, Meera, took a relieved Mataji home.

***

The very next patient Dr Rosy saw that day was one with a lax vagina. A middle-class woman and wife of a police officer, Rekha, entered her office and burst out crying. She complained that her husband was having an affair with a lady head constable. Dr Rosy was baffled.

'I am sorry, but how can I help?'

'Only you can help,' she said.

'How?! Why don't you confront *him*?'

'I did.'

'And . . .'

'And he blames me for going to another woman because, I cannot satisfy him sexually. I am so loose down there that he pulls out disgusted even if he tries to have sex with me in a drunken state. He says that he is forced to turn to another woman for a man has "needs" that I cannot satisfy.'

'Indeed! Her vagina was lax because, she had borne his children! Moreover, it could be remedied by a simple surgery, even by laser, if she could afford it. And what about a woman's needs? Why is a woman shamed and condemned if she turns to another if her husband is unable to satisfy her due to premature ejaculation or impotence?' thought Dr Rosy, her chest heaving in outrage.

After a simple surgery, Rekha's story had a happy ending. Dr Rosy saw it in her shy smile that said it all during a follow up visit. With her tightened vagina, the mother of his children now became his newly wedded bride all over again, and Rekha's husband had no need to look elsewhere.

* * *

Dr Rosy remembered the time she was a final year medical student herself, and like Rekha, had complaints quite unrelated to gynaecology.

'*Meri chat gir gaye hai* (My roof has fallen).' She had announced dramatically.

'*Bada afsoos hua, magar mere paas kyu aayi ho* (I am sorry about that but why have you come to me).'

'*Maine kaha na, meri chat gir gayi hai* (I have told you that my roof has fallen).' she repeated, as if to a moron.

On examination, Dr Rosy beheld a horrifying sight—a pink structure jutting out obscenely from her vaginal opening! On calling her senior, she had learnt that it was a case of prolapse uterus—a condition where the support that held her internal genitalia in place had indeed weakened and they had fallen out!

Dr Rosy began remembering her days in Lady Harding Hospital. After her post-graduation from AIIMS but before she started private practice, she worked as a registrar (senior resident) in this busy government hospital for a few years to gain experience. On the trusting bodies of the multitude that thronged its corridors she honed her surgical skills, and remains forever indebted to them. Whenever she saw an interesting case in the OPD, she called her junior staff, the house surgeons and the postgraduates for an on-the-spot practical class and a discussion on the diagnosis and management. Though she was a strict registrar, who brooked no nonsense, the juniors vied with each other to be posted in her unit. This was because she rewarded their hard work with the opportunity to perform major surgeries under her supervision. Most registrars would rather finish their work and rush home instead of taking on the responsibility of helping a novice perform a major surgery, besides managing the complications that occasionally arose due to their inexperience. Dr Rosy was not only kind to them when such a thing occurred, she also saw to it that the terrified young surgeon regained her/his self-confidence. It was how the complications were handled by her seniors that made or marred the confidence of a budding gynaecologist. She remembered helping a final year postgraduate perform her first vaginal hysterectomy for prolapse and was pleased to note that the student had removed the uterus vaginally quite nicely.

'You are going to be fine surgeon,' Dr Rosy told her, but she had spoken too soon. While reconstructing the loose vagina, to her horror, the postgraduate cut off a large portion of the vaginal skin! This led to a narrowing of the upper part of the vaginal canal. While the girl looked at Dr Rosy in horror, the doctor consoled her by saying, 'The vagina is a very forgiving organ, as women in general are. With a generous use of oestrogen cream, her vagina would regain its elasticity and she would be none the worse for our little misadventure.'

Coming back to the present, Dr Rosy realized that she suddenly seemed to have got a lot of such cases, even in the corporate set up. Maybe her reputation as vaginal surgeon had gone viral (no pun intended). Though she had seen more cases of prolapse uterus during her government hospital days. Prolapse of varying degree was not uncommon in the middle class and even in the upper class of the society.

It occurred chiefly due to injuries sustained during repeated vaginal births (at times, one difficult vaginal delivery was enough), but becomes more pronounced during the postmenopausal period, as tissues weaken with age and with the withdrawal of hormonal support. Some females have congenital weakness of tissue and there have been virgins with uterine prolapse!

The laxity of the genitalia that was manageable during the reproductive period, worsens after menopause and women usually come for treatment at this time. Not all cases are as severe as Mataji. Before the internal genitalia actually protrude out, women experience a dragging sensation while standing up, which can be very uncomfortable. At this stage Kegel's exercises may help and many cases do not progress beyond the manageable stage. In others, just the front part of the vagina protrudes through the vaginal opening leading to urinary complaints. Often, they have to push in the bulge to empty the bladder completely. When the posterior part of the vagina bulges, it leads to constipation and the woman must push this part in to empty her bowels completely. These are such embarrassingly peculiar problems that most women prefer to suffer in silence, when all they require is a simple surgery.

As for Mataji, Meera brought her back after a month. A vaginal surgery that entailed removing the prolapsed uterus and reconstructing the vagina was duly performed. Only after that Mataji experienced the joy of living without that 'thing' hanging out of her private parts. She realized the sufferings she had inflicted upon herself for all these years, due to misguided modesty, was unnecessary. She could only kiss Dr Rosy's hand in gratitude, hug her daughter-in-law tight and bless them both from the bottom of her heart.

Friendly advice: By the time the uterus actually prolapses out of the vagina, a woman has already been suffering unnecessarily for years. Seek medical advice when you have a bearing-down sensation or have difficult while passing urine or stool. If caught earlier, Kegels exercise and lifestyle modifications might delay/stop progress of the disease and you may not need a surgery at all.

13

HAS SHE LOST HER MIND?

A few years later, Mataji was about eighty-three years old and had lived an active, disease-free life. Except for some pain during winters, due to the wrist fractures she had suffered some years back, she had healed well enough. Life was going pretty well but Meera had been noticing of late that Mataji was withdrawing into a shell. She spoke only when spoken to and remained in her room for most of the time, even though Meera and her husband Manohar tried to get her involved in everyday activities. Even during her evening walk with their maid, she appeared lost in herself. After just one round, she would sit on a bench, gaze at the horizon with unseeing eyes and spoke not a word, whereas previously she had enjoyed interacting with people.

Matters came to a head one night when Meera was entertaining her husband's business associates for dinner. It was midnight by the time she finished washing, drying and replacing the expensive crockery that she would not trust to the maid, while her husband snored peacefully in bed, but she did not mind. In fact, she was pleased that her undemonstrative spouse had praised her culinary skills and thanked her for the effort she had put in at such short notice, because it was an important business dinner. Finally, she wiped her wet hand with the kitchen towel, removed her apron and, as was her habit, peeped into Mataji's door. She did this daily before going to bed, as she used to do with the children, when her daughters were young. To her horror, she realized that the room of this tidy old woman was in disarray and Mataji was nowhere to be found! Not in the bathroom, not in the puja room, nor anywhere else. The front door was slightly ajar, as was the gate, but wide enough to allow Mataji's frail figure to pass through! Hurriedly, she woke up her husband and the two set out to look for her. They found a dazed Mataji near the colony gate, clutching a small bag to her bosom! She was being escorted home by the guard, who knew her from her mandir days, when she would give him some prasad on the way back. The bewildered old woman had not a clue as to where she was.

Back home, addressing her son Manohar by his pet name, she said, 'Manu *beta, mainu* bus stand *chhad de. Meerut jaana hai, teri nani chal basi.* Papa *nu* phone *kar ke das de, daftar toh chutti lai kar siddhe bas adde aa jaan* (Manu, dear, drop me to the bus terminal. I have to go to Meerut for your grandmother has passed away. Ring up Papa and tell him to take leave from office and come straight to the bust terminal).'

Manohar could only stare at her in amazement. His father had expired forty years back and his maternal grandmother ten years before him! Silent tears coursed down his cheeks. What had become of his gentle mother?

In her bag, Meera found a change of clothes, a towel, a toothbrush and a comb that the poor woman had put in for her impending journey. Poor thing! Grief washed over Manohar afresh. He hugged his lost and found, yet utterly lost, mother and began to sob uncontrollably.

Her own eyes wet with tears, Mataji patted his back and consoled him, 'I know Nani loved you best of all but Manu, she was suffering so much. She is finally at peace, free from the intolerable pain.' Then pulling him away, she asked severely, 'Have you rung up your father?'

'I'm sorry, I forgot, I'll just call him up.'

The helpless couple sat with the distraught woman waiting for the morning, apparently to take Mataji to 'the bus terminal, when the bus service started'. They had pacified her with this lie while they waited to take her to the hospital. As her speech and her hands and feet movements were normal, it was not stroke or paralysis, of that they were sure; only her mind was muddled. '*Sathiya gayi hai*', as people said in crude vernacular of the old who had lost their minds.

As they waited thus, Meera related an incident that had occurred a few days back. After breakfast, Mataji usually retired to her room to read the Bhagwad Gita. That day, she reappeared after an hour and mildly admonished Meera:

'*Aj nashta dena bhul gayi* (You have forgotten to give me breakfast today)?'

'I looked at her quizzically but said nothing. When I put another plate of poha in front of her, she ate it all. Though I thought it odd, I did not tell you lest you think I was grudging your mother some extra food,' concluded Meera.

'Have you such a poor opinion of me?' asked her husband. 'Though I do not thank you enough, it isn't as if I don't see how well you treat her and with such good grace.'

Meera smiled. He usually never praised her, and this was the second time in the day! Unaware of the effect his words were having on his wife, Manohar continued, 'Mine is indeed is a happy home, with none of the *saas-bahu* quarrels one sees in most households. I only hope things remain happy.'

But it was not to be. As he learnt later from the doctor, his mother was in an advanced state of senile dementia. From now onwards, it would be a long, losing battle against the disease till the end, because there was no cure. While her mother-in-law sat huddled in a corner, totally unaware of what was going on, her son appeared as if he couldn't even move. It fell upon Meera to interact with the doctor.

'What *is* dementia?' she asked.

'It is the name given to a group of brain disorders that make it hard to remember things, think clearly, make decisions or control emotions. It also affects communication and speech, focus and attention, reasoning and judgement, which in turn impact the activities of daily life. If a person has any two of the above, it is dementia. Mataji has memory loss and lack of judgement,' concluded the doctor.

'We hear a lot about Alzheimer's these days. Are these one and the same thing?'

'Dementia is a general term for a decline in mental ability severe enough to interfere with everyday life. It usually occurs in the elderly, though it is *not* a normal part of ageing. As I told you earlier, it affects a person's ability to think, feel and communicate, thereby affecting behaviour. There are many different types of dementia and Alzheimer's is one of them. This is a specific, degenerative brain disease leading to symptoms of dementia that gradually worsens with time. The earliest symptom is difficulty in remembering new information, for the part of the brain associated with learning is impacted first.

'Dementia could also occur when clots form in the brain, stopping the blood supply to a part of the brain; this in turn affects the functioning of that particular portion. Symptoms will vary according to the part affected. Though there is no cure for any type of dementia, in cases such as these, further blood clot formation can be prevented by certain drugs. Exercise and diet also help.'

'So what do we do now?' asked Manohar.

'As your mother is frail and in a rather advanced stage of dementia, she will need a caretaker to help her with her daily activities. Encourage her to eat well and sleep well, but it will grow increasingly difficult with time. Later, she may even lose the ability to walk steadily; a fall with a fracture of the hip or the pelvis can be disastrous. Clear your house of clutter to make movements smooth and easy. The services of an occupational therapist will be required to keep her mobile. You may also need a speech therapist later. Give her a balanced, nutritious diet at short, regular intervals. With the passage of time, incontinence, severe memory loss and disorientation will slowly but surely take her down the steps to oblivion. I know I am painting a depressing picture, but I cannot give you false hope.'

'What about female hormones?' asked Meera. 'I heard that they can be of help.'

'As people age, more so women after menopause, QOL deteriorates. Some studies show that low-dose HRT significantly improves overall QOL in early menopause, but large studies found that they do not have a clinically meaningful effect later in life. Moreover, there is no reversing the damage that has already occurred.'

'QOL?'

'Quality of life,' he explained. 'WHO (World Health Organisation) defines QOL as an individual's perception of their position in life in the context of the culture and value system in which they live and in relation to their goals, expectations, standards and concerns. When the QOL pertains to health issues, it is called health-related quality of life (HRQOL). Mataji's case is advanced but there are questionnaires, like the Women's Health Questionnaire and the Menopause Rating Scale, that assess, in early stages, HRQOL in menopausal women, depending upon their symptoms.'

'I too have begun to forget things,' said Meera, alarmed. 'I stand in front of the open fridge and do not remember what I have come for. I forget where I have kept my keys and sometimes, I do not remember names. I fear that . . .' said Meera.

'Dementia isn't just about simple memory lapses. If you remember that you do not remember, you do not have dementia.'

'Thank God,' said Meera, visibly relieved, for she could not imagine her husband managing two lost women, the very women who had looked after *him* all his life.

'However, there are certain psychological changes that can occur in perimenopausal or postmenopausal women, like mood swings, memory loss, fatigue, nervousness, headaches, depression, crying spells and the inability to sleep well, but with time, most of them get over it and they lead psychologically healthy lives.'

'I have sleep disturbance,' declared Meera, who got up unrefreshed many a morning. 'I do not want to take sleeping pills lest I become addicted to them. Is there any way by which I can improve my sleep pattern?'

'Sleep disorders that include difficulty initiating and maintaining sleep are quite common in the middle-aged, but more so in the elderly. That is why a detailed assessment of menopausal symptoms includes questions about sleep pattern. You may be asked to keep a sleep diary. Adverse lifestyle factors, social factors and other risk factors contribute largely to this disorder. If there are medical or psychiatric reasons for insomnia, they are treated accordingly by the concerned specialist, as are neurological or breathing disorders.'

'But what about women who are essentially normal, like me, I hope?'

'I was coming to that. For people like you, sleep hygiene and lifestyle modifications are recommended as the first line of treatment. Psychological treatments such as Cognitive Behavioural Therapy (CBT) can also be considered if the above fail. Drugs like hypnotics can be used for a short duration, only if prescribed by psychiatrists or sleep experts.'

'I would not like to take drugs.'

'You told me so earlier. Try mind-body therapies such as yoga and meditation. They do help.'

'Sadly, we couldn't help my mother for we did not know better, but can we prevent dementia or delay its onset?' asked Manohar, glancing fleetingly at his wife.

'Memory and cognition can be best preserved in women with good overall health, which includes cardiac health. The importance of exercise and an active, occupied mind cannot be overrated. Other factors that help are reducing the risk of diabetes and hypertension, decreased intake of alcohol and no smoking.'

'If we could have recognized the condition earlier, would it have delayed the progression of the disease?'

'There is no need to blame yourself,' whispered his wife in his ear.

'I am thinking in terms of you and me,' he whispered back.

The doctor overheard every word and said, 'Dementia is a progressive disease, but early diagnosis allows a person to get the maximum benefit from available treatments and provides an opportunity to plan for the future. If only there were more memory clinics for early-stage diagnosis of dementia in India, as there are in developed countries, they would have a better prognosis. However, the plus point is that the elderly in India have a strong family support system while abroad, they have to stay in efficient but impersonal nursing homes.'

'That's true,' said Manohar, looking at his mother tenderly, though she sat still and blank as a statue, unable to register a single word.

'However, understanding each stage can help make these transitions a little easier for you and your loved one,' continued the doctor.

'Stages?'

'Stages of this progressive condition. They are as follows:

♦ Stage 1: no symptoms of cognitive (related to intellectual activity like memory, concentration, decision making, learning new things) impairment, mental function is normal.

- ◆ Stage 2: mild cognitive decline, like the typical age-related memory problems that seniors face—forgetting everyday phrases, forgetting the location of objects like keys, specs etc.
- ◆ Stage 3: where symptoms of dementia become appreciable by others, like impaired work performance, memory loss/forgetfulness, repetition of words, poor concentration, difficulty in performing complex tasks, driving etc.
- ◆ Stage 4: there is moderate cognitive decline that includes social withdrawal, moodiness, denial, non-responsiveness and trouble performing routine tasks.
- ◆ Stage 5: when people like your mother require a home caregiver or a shift to the nursing home, as they do abroad. These people are confused and forgetful, have recent memory loss and poor problem-solving capacity.

'Eventually, when your mother reaches stage 6, she will need help for Activities of Daily Living (ADLs) such as using the bathroom and eating. She may also have delusions, anxiety and difficulty recognizing loved ones and in the final stage, she may lose the ability to speak or walk.

'Though in the early stages, they manage very well on their own, for most things, assistance is required for tasks associated with memory, like doctor's appointments, help in financial matters, medications, social obligations or remembering places, people, words and names. Encourage them to maintain their independence, express their emotions, perform activities that they enjoy and establish a routine, which may delay worsening of the disease.

'The middle stages of dementia can be the longest period, but the symptoms eventually deteriorate. During this time, you will need a lot of patience and understanding, for even as you assist with everyday activities, the patient will get frustrated and angry, which can be very stressful. It is important that the caregiver unwinds with family and friends to decrease *their* stress levels.'

Dejected, Manohar and Meera took Mataji home. During the two years she survived, Mataji took her family through the entire gamut of emotions. At times, she would utter the choicest of swear words to all and sundry—the gentle lady who had not uttered a single cuss word since Meera came to her household as a daughter-in-law, but she knew them alright, as was evident now. She recollected with utter clarity an event that occurred fifty years ago, like her mother's death, but forgot what happened yesterday. Most of the time, she would not recognize anyone; at other times, she would yearn for her husband and elder son, who had died in infancy, and her sisters Kusum and Kumud. In a fit of anger, she once told Meera, 'Don't tell Papaji about my death. If he can't be with me while I live, of what use will he be to me if he comes after I am laid out on the funeral pyre? Manu can very well perform the last rites.' With tears streaming down her face, Meera could only watch helplessly.

Manohar tried to make her happy by saying, 'I got a letter from him today. He has finally got leave and is coming by the first train.' But Mataji had already retreated into her own world and cared no more.

To their horror, she disappeared once again, that too in the daytime, when Meera was in the kitchen! They found her in the park carrying a pillow in one hand and a two-rupee note in the other, asking the *maali* (gardener) directions to her beloved Meerut, where her family had lived happily for years. It was much too scary for words. An old uncle in the neighbourhood had vanished five years ago and was never found. No one knew what became of him, for people who lose their mind lose their sense of direction and almost everything else. Even if someone had found him, he would not be able to tell them the name of his family members, or his address. Thankfully, Meera and Manohar took action to prevent that for their beloved mother. Manohar kept help for her round-the-clock, who worked in two shifts of twelve hours each. Though these hired help bathed, clothed and fed her and helped with her ablutions, Meera sat with the old lady daily, whether she registered her presence or not.

Once, for a fleeting second, she recognized Meera and clung to her, crying out piteously, 'Everyone has forsaken me, promise that you will never leave me!' With tears streaming down her cheeks, Meera promised with her heart and soul, but there was no redemption for the distraught, failing old woman. Her physical woes and mental agonies aggravated as her condition deteriorated. She lost her appetite and began to wet her bed. Though diapers contained this problem, Manohar could not bear to see his mother in such a state.

When they had more or less resigned themselves to watching her decay bit by bit, one morning, premonition made Manohar go to Mataji's room at 4 a.m.—she was no more! For how long she had been like this, no one knew, because the night help had dozed off. Though heartbroken, Manohar was relieved that his mother's suffering was over.

Menopausal quote: Welcome to the age where your secrets are safe with your friends ... they can't remember them either.

14

THE BEAUTY AND HER BREAST

Today, the ladies gathered in the seminar room at Mascot Enterprises were wary. Dr Rosy was going to discuss the breast—a thing of beauty, joy, utility and fear. She breezed in like a breath of fresh air and began in a merry, sing-song voice:

'We flash them, we smash them
We push them way up
We shake them we stuff them
In the wrong-sized cup
Our husbands just crave them
Our children have drained them
Some of us even decided to name them
We go through our lives and knock them about
But one thing is certain, one thing I must shout
Our boobies have been there through thick
and through thin
And life is too precious to let cancer win.

'I do not know who wrote this poem, but it is apt. Women spare no effort to accentuate their contours and deepen their cleavage, but do not spare a moment to feel them for lumps, which is a sorry state of affairs indeed. Despite the mischievous poem I just recited, I would like to tell you right at the outset, do not expect this talk to be humorous, for I find nothing funny about breast cancer. Please listen carefully to what I have to say, learn what I have to teach and, in turn, teach what I have taught to every single woman you know so that we do our bit to decrease the incidence of breast cancer in our country.'

The ladies looked at each other, perplexed. They had never seen this aspect of Dr Rosy's personality—a fiery crusader against breast cancer. Caught in the sway, they were quite willing to join the crusade and waited for Dr Rosy to tell them what to do.

Continuing her tirade, directed towards husbands this time, Dr Rosy said, 'No other part of a woman's body has been so eulogized as her breasts. Even centuries earlier, Sanskrit poets were not immune to its beauty. Shakuntala's nipples were likened to bumblebees and Krishna is supposed to have painted on Radha's breasts! As for our menfolk, they fondle and handle breasts, derive exquisite pleasure from them, but surprisingly, fail to detect a lump during foreplay, for a clinical examination is the last thing on their minds at that time.

'What I want to impress upon your minds is that the breast, which gives so much pleasure to man and woman alike, the breast that sustains a child during infancy, is also a potential source of dread and death. Breast cancer is the most common cancer in females the world over. Though it was second only to cancer of the cervix in India till recently, it is fast catching up in the race to become the no. 1 killer here too. It is a disease of urbanization, being three times higher in cities than in rural India, and has already overtaken cervical cancer in metropolises in many parts of India'

'What has urbanization to do with it?' asked Mona perplexed.

'Women in cities have a higher socio-economic status, increased income and a higher education level.'

'So? I still don't understand what that has to do with breast cancer.'

'Due to the above advantages, women to lead a sedentary lifestyle, with lower levels of physical activity, an unhealthy dietary pattern and hence suffer from obesity. The obstetric history (history of childbirths) of a woman in the city too is vastly different from that of her rural counterparts. She tends to have early menarche (first period), late menopause (the more a woman is exposed to female sex hormones, the higher is the chance of developing breast cancer), marries late, delays childbearing, forgoes breastfeeding and limits the number of children, all of which are contributory factors, while village women work hard, eat less, marry early, have a number of offspring and breastfeed them though early initiation of sex life, multiple partners and poor sexual hygiene increases the risk of cervical cancer (cancer of the mouth of the womb) in these women. There are other factors that predispose a woman to breast cancer, but we will come to those later.'

'Yes, please,' said Mona thoughtfully.

'And that is not all. According to Breast Cancer India (BCI), breast cancer develops at least ten years earlier in Indian woman As compared to their Western counter parts accounting for 37.7 per cent of cancers between the age group of 25–49 years. To put matter in perspective, BCI highlights a horrific fact—one Indian woman is diagnosed with breast cancer every 4 minutes and one woman in India woman dies of breast cancer, every 8 minutes!

The numbers are staggering and constantly rising. What fills me with anger is that the breast is such an accessible organ and breast cancer is such a preventable cause of death! As this master killer is painless in the initial stages, dangerous lumps are missed or ignored. When the pain becomes evident eventually, it is already too late. A single-digit addition to the cancer mortality statistics may seem insignificant, but the devastation wrought by the death of a young woman with a young family that needs her desperately is beyond words! And yes, men too can develop breast cancer! Though it is rare in them, it spreads faster.'

Seeing that she had her audience riveted to her talk, Dr Rosy went on, 'Breast cancer is a treatable disease and chances of survival are much higher *if* it is detected in time, but sadly, in India, **detection is late.** The only way to increase the early detection rate is by increasing awareness and there is where **you** come in, but let me begin at the beginning.

'Cancer of the breast has modifiable and non-modifiable risk factors. As we can do nothing about the latter, we will have to focus on modifying the modifiable factors.

Non-Modifiable Risk Factors
◆ Age
◆ Family history
◆ Benign breast disease (lumps or breast condition that are non-cancerous)
◆ BRCA 1 or 2 gene mutation (which I will discuss later)

♦ Early menarche (<twelve years), late age at menopause (after age fifty-five)
♦ Increased breast density as seen on mammography (X-ray of the breast soft tissue)

Modifiable Risk Factors
♦ Age at first child
♦ Breastfeeding
♦ Parity (number of children)
♦ Obesity
♦ Physical activity
♦ HRT (Hormone Replacement Therapy) can lead to a slight increase the incidence of breast cancer.
♦ Diet and lifestyle choices: smoking, alcohol, high fat diet
♦ Radiation Exposure: Frequent exposure to X-Rays and CT scans

As for prevention of breast cancer, the crux of today's talk, you could begin by:

Prevention Of Breast Cancer
♦ Adopting a healthy lifestyle
♦ Maintaining optimal weight
♦ Breastfeeding
♦ Being aware of family cancer history and taking preventive measures
♦ Breast self-examination (BSE) every month from the twenties onwards

'BSE is what I am going to teach you in detail and ask you to teach every other female you come across so that she can teach all *her* female contacts. Understood?'

'Yes, ma'am,' they chorused like children in a classroom, which made her smile for the first time.

'Now, coming to the most important part of today's discussion...

BSE (Breast Self-Examination)

It is performed by the woman herself, during which she sees and feels her breast from her armpit to her bra line. It is initially done frequently during the entire month so that she understands the usual changes that occur in a breast during the menstrual cycle, and the nodular lumpy feel just before her periods does not alarm her. Once she is familiar with the normal, it will become easier for her to detect the abnormal later on. Thereafter, BSE is done every month, a day or two after her periods end. Pregnant or postmenopausal women can select a particular day each month to do a BSE. It should not be performed in the shower or with lotion on your skin or fingers. Report any recent or persistent changes to the doctor. If you do find a lump, do not panic. About 80 per cent of lumps are non-cancerous, but visit a doctor promptly for further evaluation. Is there anyone who is brave enough to volunteer? I will be showing you exactly how it is done.'

Thirty-four-year-old Reema, who was anyway fond of showing off her magnificent figure with clingy skirts and blouses with deep décolletage, stepped forwards. As instructed, she took off her blouse and bra quite unselfconsciously. Might as well get a free check-up now.

'For once, she is showing them for a good cause,' thought the envious Mala.

'Thank you, Reema. BSE involves two steps:

- ♦ Visual inspection—look
- ♦ Palpation—feel

Visual inspection

Stand in front of a mirror and look at your breasts from the front, right and left sides, standing straight with your arms by your side, then raise your arms above your head, and finally, with hands on your hips and hunched forward.

Check for:

- ♦ Size and shape: one breast is usually larger than the other or lower, but look for sudden changes in size or shape
- ♦ Redness
- ♦ Puckering
- ♦ Rash
- ♦ Orange peel appearance of the skin
- ♦ Increase in the size and number of veins in one breast compared to the other.
- ♦ Examine the nipples for
  - o retraction (drawing inwards)
  - o redness
  - o scaliness
  - o discharge

Palpation

To feel **the outer part of your right breast,** lie down and turn slightly to your left side by placing a pillow under your shoulder and back. This way, your breast will be on your chest and not slide laterally as it does while lying down flat. Raise your right hand, palm upwards, and start feeling your breast from your armpit using the flat (not the tip) of the middle three fingers of your left hand, making small rotatory motions. The pressure should be mild first, then moderate and finally deep, so that the entire depth of that part of the breast is palpated for lumps. Making similar little circles, go right down to the bottom of your breast, down to the bra line. Move your hand a finger breadth medially and slide it up to repeat the circular movement with varying pressure till you again reach the bottom. Do this till the entire outer half of the breast has been palpated.

Once you reach the nipple, remove the pillow and place the right arm at right angles to your body. Carefully feel the nipple area for any abnormalities. Follow this up with an examination of the inner half of your breast, like you examined the outer half. Repeat the same procedure with the other breast. There are a number of videos on the net which you can observe and follow. Here are a couple of links:

https://www.nationalbreastcancer.org/breast-self-exam
https://youtu.be/UyePcbnoOLQ

Other methods that are done by the doctors are:

- ♦ Clinical breast exams (CBE) every three years, starting in the twenties till the age of thirty-nine, and annually thereafter.
- ♦ Mammographic screening (annually) starting at the age of forty years.

CBE (Clinical Breast Examination)

For women between fifty and seventy years of age, annual CBE is a must. It is performed by the clinician, who checks all the four quadrants of the breast, the nipple, the part of the breast called the axillary tail, which extends into the armpit, and the area above the collarbone, with the flat of her hand. She will look for lumps, skin changes, nipple retraction and discharge.

Broadly speaking, benign breast lumps like fibroadenomas are well-circumscribed and firm mass(es). A fibroadenoma is so freely mobile that is it called a 'mouse in the breast'. Cancer usually appears as an irregular, hard, painless lump, but these are generalizations and every breast lump has to be investigated thoroughly.

Mammogram

This is an X-ray of the soft tissue of the breast. Though someone joked 'this is the only time you will be filmed topless at this age' it is no laughing matter. It is slightly painful, for the breast tissue is compressed from above downwards and from side to side between two X Ray plates to get films from all views. As breast cancer incidence peaks before the age of fifty years in India, a mammography is usually done after forty years of age, or even before, in those with suspicious breast lesions. When the breast tissue appears dense on mammography, the patient is usually sent for ultrasound of both breasts (also called sonomammography), and if an abnormal mass is found, FNAC (fine needle aspiration), or better still, a true cut biopsy is taken for histopathological confirmation of diagnosis.

PET (Positron Emission Tomography) scan has a limited role in breast cancer due to its low sensitivity and is used only to see if chemotherapy is working or not. I have given it a passing reference just to get it out of the way.

MRI is done along with mammography in high-risk patients, which includes BRCA 1 or 2 mutation carriers.

This brings us to the most famous case in the world associated with BRCA gene testing and breast cancer prevention—that of actress and sex symbol Angelina Jolie. That she decided to get rid of her beautiful breasts at the age of thirty-seven (and later, her ovaries too) because of BRCA 1 gene mutation, became an issue of international import. Suddenly, there was large-scale interest in testing for BRCA 1 and 2 gene mutation. She went public with her decision to take such drastic measures for cancer prevention, so that other women in a similar situation learn about it and make an informed choice.

In an op-ed for *The New York Times* in April 2013), she said that she decided to do what she did after doctors told her that she carried a "faulty gene" that increased the chances of her developing breast cancer by about 87 per cent risk besides carrying 50 per cent risk of developing ovarian cancer. Her mother died of ovarian and breast cancer when she was just 56 years old. Her grandmother and aunt also died from cancer. After mastectomy her chances of developing breast cancer dropped to under 5 per cent! In another op-ed for The New York Times in March 2015, she revealed she had her ovaries and fallopian tubes removed to reduce the chances of developing ovarian cancer. Though, this surgery was simpler, it led to premature menopause.

Suddenly enormous interest was generated in testing for BRCA 1 and 2 gene mutation but, a Harvard Medical School study, published 14 December in The BMJ, revealed that the large spike in genetic testing for breast cancer risk following Jolie's op-ed, did not show a corresponding rise mastectomy (breast removal) rates, suggesting the tests did not lead to increased breast cancer diagnoses. This was because women in the low-risk group too got themselves tested in large numbers.

Now, what is this test all about? BRCA 1 and BRCA 2 genes maintain the stability of a cell's genetic material, called DNA, and help prevent uncontrolled cell growth. Mutation of these genes has been linked to the development of hereditary breast and ovarian cancer and occurs in individuals with a personal or family history of cancer— first, second or third-degree relative, maternal or paternal— which occurs at a younger age as compared to their non-hereditary counterparts. About 13 per cent of women in the general population will develop breast cancer sometime during their lives. By contrast, 55–72 per cent of women who inherit a harmful *BRCA 1* variant and 45–69 per cent of women who inherit a harmful *BRCA 2* variant will develop breast cancer by 70–80 years of age.

The risk of contralateral breast cancer increases, reaching 20–30 per cent at 10 years of follow-up and 40–50 per cent at 20 years.

Ovarian cancer: About 1.2 per cent of women in the general population will develop ovarian cancer sometime during their lives. By contrast, 39–44 per cent of women who inherit a harmful *BRCA 1* variant and 11–17 per cent of women who inherit a harmful *BRCA 2* variant will develop ovarian cancer by 70–80 years of age.*

---

*https://www.cancer.gov/about-cancer/causes-prevention/genetics/brcafact-sheet

BRCA 1 and 2 gene testing should be done in case there is:

♦ A personal history of breast or ovarian cancer diagnosed at a young age (premenopausal) or below the age of forty-five
♦ Bilateral breast cancer (affecting both breasts)
♦ Occurrence of both ovarian and breast cancer in the same woman or the same family
♦ A family history of breast, ovarian, fallopian tube, peritoneal, prostate or pancreatic cancer
♦ A male family member having breast cancer
♦ A relative with a known BRCA 1 or BRCA 2 gene mutation
♦ A family member with bilateral breast cancer below the age of fifty
♦ Two or more relatives with ovarian cancer
♦ Jewish ethnicity as Ashkenazi Jewish women have 1:40 risk of gene mutation
♦ Non-hormone-dependent breast cancers*

*As we have seen, women on HRT (specially progesterone) have a slightly higher risk of developing breast cancer, but whether a breast cancer is hormone-dependent or not is confirmed by certain tests. A triple-negative breast cancer is not hormone dependent.

'Medical jargon aside, there are certain medical conditions that warrant a BRCA gene testing, and the doctor will prescribe it if indicated. The test costs about Rs 20,000 to Rs 23,000 in India and the result is available in two to three weeks. A negative report brings with it a sense of relief, though one must never be lax about regular check-ups, for the price of neglect will be too heavy to pay. Those with a positive BRCA report can make an informed choice regarding the removal of their breasts and ovaries. Those who do not opt for surgery have to come for rigorous follow-up so that when the cancer does occur, it is caught early.

Breast cancer prevention

The risk of breast cancer may be lowered largely by the following:

- Lifestyle changes as follows:
  o maintain optimal weight
  o physical activity: must be a part of your routine
  o eat the right type of food in the right quantity at the right time
  o judicious use of HRT under medical supervision, if at all
  o have your first child early
  o breastfeed your children
  o parityin family. This one thing I cannot ask you to do—increase the number of children to decrease the incidence of breast cancer
- Breast self-examination every month
- Clinical breast examination
- Mammography
- MRI in select cases
- BRCA 1 and 2 gene testing in high-risk population
- Risk-reducing surgery, mastectomy, salpingo-oophorectomy (removal of tubes and ovaries) after discussion with experts. The decision is individualized.

'Got it, girls?'

'Yes!'

'I hope that I have managed to convince you all that breast cancer is preventable and treatable to a large extent, if diagnosed early. Despite this, women die of this dreadful disease every day. It is in a mad race to overtake cervix cancer as the primary cause of cancer mortality in our country and has already done so in the urban population. What is just a number in the statistical register could spell devastation for an entire family, for the woman is the pivot around which it revolves. It is indeed a very sorry state of affairs, but we can and must add our mite to decrease the numbers. Will you help me to do so?'

'Yes, we definitely will.'

'At the cost of repetition, I want to impress upon you the importance of breast self-examination, which you all will do once a month (after your periods if menstruating) and teach it to each and every female you come across, be it your maid or your child's teacher, even your boss. You will

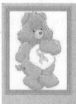

Breast Cancer Awareness

If you see these 'Little Pink Ribbons',
On sale within a store...
Please take the time to buy one,
And say Breast Cancer "NO MORE"...

In loving memory of 'Women Gone',
And those suffering today...
All the women of our future,
May a 'cure' be found - we pray...

© Mary G - Love for All

be doing yourself and the nation a favour by preventing the loss of lives due to such a preventable cause of death. Are you motivated enough to do so?'

'Yes!' they chorused, visibly moved.

'Finally, I want to show you something.'

'Do you see the pink ribbon in this picture? It is an international symbol of breast cancer awareness and means that the wearer is either a patient with breast cancer or expresses moral support for women with breast cancer. And I agree totally with the little poem written alongside.

Friendly advice: Breast self-examination every month is a must. Do not ignore any breast lump however small or painless.

15

RAMA, A LOST CAUSE?

Rama woke up to a flurry of kisses. His lips, light as a feather, were on her forehead, then her closed eyelids, the tip of her nose, her neck, the angles of her mouth, building up to finally find her lips and pull her into a kiss, hard and long. Her husband Rajat had returned from a two-month deputation abroad and had made passionate love to her last night. Naked and replete, they had slept in each other's arms. In the morning, he was at it again, but in a more relaxed manner, savouring every bit of her luscious, responsive flesh. Down he slid to curl his tongue around the nipple of her left breast as he held the plump right one in his large hand, his male hardness pressing against her. Her body ached for him and she parted her thighs with delicious anticipation. Just as he was about to enter her, he stopped short. It was as if someone had doused his ardour with a bucket of cold water.

'Are you having your periods?' he asked.

'No, they are not due for another week,' she said, sliding up from under him to see the blood on the sheet beneath her.

Perhaps the vigorous sex they had the previous night led to the initiation of menstruation a week earlier, she thought, but to her surprise, the bleeding lasted for just a day and she had her periods exactly a week later, at the right time. They had abstained from sex in the interim but when they tried again after a fortnight, she bled again. When this threatened to become a pattern, they stopped having sex altogether. She knew that this was not the remedy for her malady but was too embarrassed to discuss the issue with anyone. Now she had begun spotting off and on even between periods, without provocation, and was at her wits' end. The stress began to tell on her, making her moody and withdrawn. The sombre look did not become her, for she had a bubbly personality with a ready laugh. When her sister-in-law Reena tried to draw her out, she evaded the issue, but could hold back only for so long. The dam burst and her shameful secret tumbled out, along with her tears.

'How long has this been going on, Didi?' asked Reena, alarmed.

'Since Rajat returned from abroad, about four months.'

'And you have done nothing about it?'

'What could I do except stop having sex?'

'That's not the solution.'

'Then what is?'

'Let's consult Dr Rosy tomorrow.' They had known her since she had operated upon their mother-in-law Shiela and liked her very much.

So the next morning, after sending the menfolk off to work, the kids to school and mom-in-law to the nursery school she ran, the two met the good doctor. She listened to them gravely, sent Reena out and examined Rama gently.

Post-coital (after sex) bleeding could be the first sign of cancer of the cervix (mouth of the uterus), though there could be other causes for the same, like a cervical polyp, a bad cervical erosion, infections and, rarely, TB of the cervix.

It was as she had feared all along. An ominous, small cauliflower-like growth that bled on touch stared at her from the cervix when she did a speculum examination. In all probability, it was cancer of the cervix, but a biopsy would be diagnostic. Of course, she did not want to scare the girls right now, though she did impress upon them the urgent need for a biopsy; only after the histopathology report would she be able to give an accurate diagnosis.

Alarmed, the two women went home and told their family what had happened. The very next day, Maaji and Rajat went with Rama to the hospital while Reena managed the house and their kids. The biopsy itself was a minor procedure, though the bleeding was slightly more than expected. This, too, went in favour of the cervix cancer diagnosis, but Dr Rosy refrained from giving her opinion till she had confirmatory evidence.

The days between the biopsy and the report passed with excruciating slowness. Finally, the trio was again seated in Dr Rosy's office, looking at her as to a hangman, begging for redemption, which she could not give. The grave look on the face of the jovial doctor did nothing to allay their fears. Dr Rosy looked at the report and then at Rama, compassion writ large across her face. There was no way one could break such news gently. This was something that was not taught in medical college and though she had been imparting bad news for years, she was still not comfortable doing it. There were times when she had to tell a couple that they would never be able to have a baby, a pregnant woman that her baby had died inside her womb or was abnormal, a husband that his wife had died of massive haemorrhage after delivery, leaving behind a wailing motherless child, but worst of all was telling someone that she had cancer. The very word evoked such dread that the patient went either into shock or denial. No matter how much she tried to tell them that cancer was not what it was, say, twenty years ago; that with better treatment modalities, life expectancy had increased greatly, as had the quality of life; the sense of doom it evoked was difficult to overcome.

Needless to say, this family too was stunned by the news. No matter how hard she tried to soften the blow by saying that as it was in the early stage, the chances of a cure were very good, the only word that reverberated through Rama's brain was 'cancer', 'cancer', 'cancer'. It chilled her to the bone and squeezed the blood from her heart with icy fingers. She was just forty-three years old and did not want to die. What would become of her children? They were so young—her son eighteen and daughter sixteen! No matter how much her husband loved her, he would marry again after she died. And her children would be at the mercy of a stepmother. And the pain—she had heard that people with cancer had unbearable pain towards the end. She had not even been able to bear labour pains and had opted for painless labour with epidural anaesthesia both times. Could she now opt for a painless death or would she have to kill herself to avoid the pain? Such morbid thoughts scurried around like rats in her skull, gnawing at her brain, and she broke down completely. Though her husband put his arm around her and moved his hand up and down her shoulder to console her, he too looked stunned beyond comprehension. Only Shiela, the middle-aged matron who had braved the vagaries of life over the years, wore a look of stoic resignation. Shiela told Rajat to take Rama outside, for she had matters to discuss with the doctor.

'Why does it occur?' was the first question she posed after the two had left.

'Cervical cancer, for that matter, any cancer, occurs when healthy cells in the cervix develop changes (mutations) in their DNA. A cell's DNA contains instructions that tell a cell what to do. Healthy cells grow and multiply at a set rate and eventually die at a set time. The mutation tells the cells to grow and multiply out of control, and they don't die. The accumulating abnormal cells form a mass (tumour). As the cancer progresses, malignant cells invade nearby tissues and finally spread (metastasize) to distant organs through the blood stream or the lymphatic system.'

'Could it have been diagnosed earlier?'

'Early-stage cervical cancer generally produces no signs or symptoms. Rama has come early enough though she could have come four months back, when she first noticed the symptom, but most women are too embarrassed to discuss such an issue.'

Dr Rosy showed her a model of cervical cancer that she held in her hand.

Cancer cervix

'What information has the biopsy provided?'

'The biopsied tissue was sent to the lab for histopathology examination (HPE). HPE is the gold standard in diagnosing cancer, its type and the extent of its invasion into the deeper tissues. This has a bearing on the prognosis and treatment modality. In Rama's case, it has confirmed the diagnosis of cancer cervix, given information regarding its type—squamous cell carcinoma (which is the commonest variety)—and reported that it has not invaded deeply, which is a good sign.'

'Now what?'

'Now we will stage the cancer, i.e., delineate the extent of its spread in the uterus, the adjoining organs like the rectum and bladder, and to distant organs like the liver and lungs. She will be sent for an X-ray, CT, MRI and PET scan to determine whether the cancer has spread beyond the cervix. The lesser the spread, the better is the five-year survival rate.'

'Five-year survival?'

'That is how the life expectancy of a patient with cancer is measured—the lower the stage, the higher the percentage of five-year survival. That does not mean that a person with cancer survives for a maximum of five years. When it is caught early, the patient becomes completely cancer-free and lives a healthy, productive life.'

'I hope and pray that Rama is one of them.'

'Clinically, she appears to be one of them, but let's hurry up with the tests so that treatment can be started at the earliest.'

'Yes.'

'Another thing: from now on, an oncologist will be her primary caretaker.' On seeing the look of alarm on Shiela's face, the doctor pacified her by adding, 'I will continue to play an active part by assisting them in the surgery and daily postoperative visits.'

'Please do, doctor. We are counting on you.'

'I am not forsaking her, only handing her over to the expert in this field. I will personally introduce you to a very efficient and compassionate oncologist. The plan of action will be discussed by the medical/surgical oncologist and the radiotherapist in a tumour board meeting. They will go through the test reports and decide which treatment option is best for her. At times, two or even all three modalities have to be combined to obtain optimal results.'

'That means the treatment could be long-drawn and demoralizing.'

'This is where the counsellor and family come in—a strong family support system is of the utmost importance. You all have the extremely important task of keeping her morale high; it makes all the difference between the success and failure of a treatment. If cancer falls in the bad company of gangsters like dread, depression and despair, it will drag her down. Instead, give her hope, faith and lots of love, which will boost her immunity and the cancer will slink away, tail between its legs. Keep her spirits high in whatever way possible—religion, meditation, yoga—but best of all is TLC (tender loving care).'

'That we surely will, doctor. Ours is a close-knit joint family and she is as dear as a daughter to me.'

Her first bout of grief expended somewhat, Rama and her husband were called back into her office and given a brief summary of what Dr Rosy had explained in detail to Shiela.

'I will now entrust you to the care of Dr Pandit, a genitourinary oncologist who has gained considerable repute as a laparoscopic oncologist. Rama's recovery will be quick if her operation can be done by minimally invasive surgery, which I know is possible, considering the stage, but let the oncologist decide what is best for her.'

Soon, Rama found herself on the operation table, smiling back at the tall, lanky Dr Pandit, with his infectious smile and an efficient manner that made her trust him implicitly. On her other side stood Dr Rosy, holding her hand. With the two of them by her side, Rama was ready to take on her cancer and thumb her nose at it. It was the attitude of the patient that made all the difference between the success and failure of a treatment and after the initial show of weakness, she had composed herself reasonably well. She had but one question to ask Dr Rosy: 'Will I live long enough to see my children educated and settled?'

'Of course; and keep this in mind—I will be coming for both their marriages, whether you invite me or not.'

'Is that a promise?'

'Yes, it is.'

To see her children educated and married became the goal she clung to, the one thing that made her want to get the better of her cancer. Drawing on reserves of strength that she did not know she possessed, Rama had decided that she would live, and there was nothing that the cancer or anything else could do about it. So there!

The operation went off without a hitch. As she was young, medically fit and her cancer had been caught in the early stage, her prognosis was good. Rama's family took turns to sit by her during her hospital stay. Rajat did not want to leave her side, but he was forced to go home and rest; moreover, his children needed him now more than ever. When it was Reena's turn and Rama was deeply asleep after sedation, she went downstairs to Dr Rosy's OPD for a consult. Now that there was one woman with cancer in the family, and a dear one at that, Reena needed to know if there were ways of preventing it.

'Yes,' replied Dr Rosy, 'there are. How old are you?'

'Thirty-seven years.'

'There are two things that you can do. Get yourself vaccinated against HPV virus and get a Pap smear and HPV testing done every year. If you follow what I say diligently, rest assured, you will not get cancer cervix. If at all a precancerous lesion is detected, it can be dealt with by simple procedures, years before it can become cancerous.'

'What is HPV and how does a vaccine against HPV help?'

'Though other factors, like early initiation of sexual activity, multiple sex partners, multiple deliveries, tobacco, low socio-economic status, poor local hygiene and long-term use of hormonal contraceptives can lead to cancer cervix, HPV is the single most important contributing factor. HPV (Human Papilloma Virus) is a sexually transmitted virus. There are many strains of HPV, but serotypes 16 and 18 account for nearly 76.7 per cent of cervical cancer in India.* The other strains cause vaginal warts, but the strains responsible for changes in the cervix that eventually lead to cancer cause no symptoms. Sadly, condoms do **not** offer protection because the infection spreads by skin-to-skin contact.'

'And how does the HPV vaccine help?'

'It takes fifteen to twenty years for a patient with **persistent** (though there is no treatment for HPV, it is

---

*https://www.ncbi.nlm.nih.gov/pmc/articles/PMC3385284/#

cleared naturally from the genital tract of healthy young women, hence the term persistent) infection with oncogenic (cancer-causing) HPV strains to develop cancer. Keeping this in mind, a vaccine against HPV was developed to prevent cervical cancer. It induces a strong protective immune response, preventing the virus from releasing its genetic material. The two vaccines licensed globally, Gardasil and Cervirax, are freely available in India.'

'Can I get vaccinated now?'

'Yes, it is recommended for all females between the ages of nine and forty-five, as cancer cervix is the commonest cancer in India and a preventable one. However, it will not protect against the strain a patient is already infected with, hence, the trick is to catch them young. The ideal time to vaccinate a girl is before she has made her sexual debut, the recommended age being between nine and twelve years.'

'My daughter is twelve years old and Didi's daughter is sixteen.'

'You must get them vaccinated too. It is the best age. Tell your friends, who in turn should tell their friends, to get all the females they know in this age group vaccinated. Abroad, they are vaccinating boys too, which is a good step in carrying the cancer cervix eradication program still further.'

'And in India?'

'The government is working towards it.'

'I want to clarify one thing. If I am already infected by a carcinogenic strain, I will not be protected against it.'

'Yes, but it is still useful, so do get vaccinated for protection against other strains.'

'Is there a way of knowing if I have the infection?'

'Yes, but we'll come to that later. Let's complete the vaccination part first. It has to be given in a total of three doses in the following manner:

| Dosage Schedule In Months ||
Gardasil	Cervirax
0	0
2	1
6	6

'The vaccine is administered in the upper arm and the patient should be observed for 15 minutes for the rare possibility of a fainting attack. It can be given simultaneously with other vaccines such as Hepatitis B. Side effects could take the form of mild to moderate pain, swelling and redness at the site of injection.'

'Is a booster required later?

'Follow-up studies have shown no evidence of waning immunity and no booster is required. If the HPV vaccine schedule is interrupted, the vaccine series need not be restarted. If interrupted after the first dose, the second dose should be administered as soon as possible, with an interval of at least twelve weeks between the second and third doses. If only the third dose is delayed, it should be administered as soon as possible.

'The vaccine should be deferred in patients with moderate or severe acute illnesses. It is **not** recommended in pregnant women. Feeding mothers can receive it,' concluded Dr Rosy.

'I will bring the girls and get myself vaccinated along with them as soon as possible.'

'Good. Now coming to the next part of the prevention programme, a Pap smear. Though the vaccine is a giant leap forward in preventing cancer cervix, it is not foolproof for, as I have told you earlier, there are other causes of cancer cervix. So all sexually active woman should get a yearly Pap smear done. It is a painless OPD procedure during which the doctor scrapes and brushes cells from your cervix, which are then examined in a lab for abnormal cells. LBC (liquid-based cytology) is a better version of Pap smear and is done along with HPV DNA testing in high resource set-ups like ours. If dysplastic (abnormal) changes are seen in the report, you do not have to panic because firstly, it could be due to anything, from infection to erosion to precancerous changes. HPV also causes changes in Pap smear, ranging from low-grade to high-grade precancerous lesions that finally end in cancer cervix, but as we have caught them years before they could become cancerous, we have **simple remedies for a complete cure**. There are procedures like colposcopy (which gives a magnified view of the cervix), during which the cervix is painted with dyes like ascetic acid or Lugol's iodine, which highlight suspicious areas from which a biopsy is taken. These lesions are treated with minimal surgical procedures like cryosurgery, cautery or conization.'

'My head is reeling, but I got the gist.'

'I'm sorry to confuse you with medical jargon. We'll cross that bridge when we come to it, which hopefully we will not. Meanwhile, the message I want you to take home is get a Pap smear/LBC done every year, even if you are fully vaccinated.'

'Yes, ma'am. Can I get it done now?'

'Yes, if you have not had an internal examination or sexual intercourse in the last twenty-four hours.'

'No,' said Reena, thinking, where was the mood or inclination for sexual enjoyment when gloom loomed like a pall overhead?

'Now, coming to the part that is worrying you—how will you know if you are already infected with the cancer-causing strain of HPV? The very cells taken on a brush for Pap smear can be simultaneously sent for HPV DNA testing, as I will be doing in your case. If it is positive for carcinogenic strains of HPV, **do not panic.** Come for follow-up testing at six to twelve months intervals for, as I have already told you, our immune system gets rid of the virus in most cases. Only those with persistent infection need diligent monitoring.'

'I see.'

'If Rama had got these done, her condition could have been caught in the precancerous stage and treated completely before it actually turned into cancer. That window period is lost to her, but it is still available to you and thousands of women out there.'

'Poor Didi.'

'She is far better off than others for her cancer was caught early. With improved surgical techniques and newer treatment modalities, she has a good chance of living a long, healthy life.'

'I sincerely hope so,' said Reena, sending out a prayer.

'Once she recovers from her illness, I want both of you to become active crusaders for cancer prevention. Will you do that for the other women out there whose lives can be saved by your efforts? Cervical cancer is the fifth most common cancer in humans, the second most common cancer in women worldwide and the most common cancer in women in India (though breast cancer is fast catching up).

Just think of the number of lives you will be able to save by motivating women to get HPV vaccination and a Pap smear done.'

'Yes.'

'It is such a wonderful feeling, to be able to save a life. We doctors are blessed for our profession gives us the opportunity to do so time and again. Now you too have the chance to become God's agent on earth. Will you be one?'

Reena nodded her head vigorously, too choked with emotion to utter a word.

Friendly advice: HPV vaccination and regular PAP smear/HPV DNA testing will drastically decrease the chances of getting cervical cancer. Immediately report to your doctor if there is post coital-bleeding, bleeding/spotting in between periods and blood stained vaginal discharge.

16

MENOPAUSAL MAPPING OF THE SKIN

'Is there a system in our body that menopause does not affect?' Dr Rosy asked her female audience when she met them next in the seminar room at Mascot Enterprises.

'None,' came the emphatic answer.

'Sadly, I agree. Today, I am going to talk about the various ways in which it stamps its presence on our skin, that too in capital letters. Did you know that the skin is the largest organ of our body?'

They looked as each other, surprised. At the most, if they ever thought of the skin, it was as a covering of their body, but an organ?

'Though the effect of female hormone depletion on skin and hair is not as devastating as its effect on the heart, bones and genitourinary systems,' continued Dr Rosy, 'it is the most visible evidence of ageing; the one that worries a woman most. Why? Because is it like a banner broadcasting her age. Now, why a woman wants to look younger than she is is something I won't dwell upon. On second thoughts, I *will* touch upon it in passing. I think it is due to the western influence, which sets such store by youth, that our urban population strives to look young. This has given birth to a thriving anti-ageing industry. Creams for a wrinkle-free skin that flood the market have the same effect as 'fair and lovely' creams have on dark skin—none. Better to invest in a healthy lifestyle with adequate amounts of exercise, sleep and the right type of food, and strive for mental peace with yoga and meditation. You will glow with an inner radiance that no beauty products can bestow. Our grandmothers, with their homemade non-toxic beauty products like besan and *malai*, physical labour and regular eating and sleeping habits fared much better than us, with our stressful, ambitious lives, late-night parties, binging, drinking, smoking and insomnia, which is reflected in our dull, lifeless skins: flaws that concealers are unable to conceal.

'Indian women in the hinterland, not touched by the West, are comfortable in their skins, even if they are old and wrinkled. My maid talks fondly of her granny, who looked after her when her mother died. She was totally unselfconscious of her wrinkled face, loose underarms that jiggled with every movement and hanging breasts that she could flip over her shoulders. Despite her skin being two sizes big for her, the old lady was wiry and fit, worked as hard as anyone else and that was what mattered at the end of the day.

'As you age, which skin changes do you fear the most?' Dr Rosy threw an open question to the house.

'Wrinkles!' nearly all said unanimously.

'The thinning of scalp hair and the appearance of facial hair,' said Surbhi in horror.

'Moles sprouting hair and an outcrop of warts, as I saw on someone,' said Mala.

'You really are a mean lot!' said Dr Rosy, laughing.

'I know is bad to talk like this, but why didn't they do something about it?' asked Mala.

'Maybe it didn't bother them; maybe they didn't know that something *could* be done about it. Our generation knows better. Any other skin changes you have seen in the ageing female population?'

'Dryness and age spots.'

'Okay girls, enough. You have summarized menopausal skin changes beautifully, except for a few things. Let me round off the list. Around fifty years of age, the pH level of our skin changes, making it sensitive. This could lead to rashes and skin irritation. Pre-existing skin conditions may worsen. Also, at this age, one becomes more prone to precancerous skin conditions and skin cancer. Most of the skin changes occur in the first five years after menopause, after which they slow down.'

'Thank heaven for small mercies,' said a cheeky voice from the back.

Ignoring the comment, Dr Rosy asked, 'And why does it happen?'

'Due to depletion of female hormones,' sang a few bored voices together. They were fed up hearing the same thing over and over again.

'It seems to be the root of all evil,' said someone petulantly.

'Agreed, but you do not have to have such a defeatist attitude. I am sure you must have come across many postmenopausal women who have aged gracefully and look beautiful, like Sharmila Tagore.'

'Like you,' said Mona loyally.

'Thanks,' said Dr Rosy, smiling. 'If you think you are going to change from beauties into witches without their brooms with age, let me tell you, that depends largely upon you. If you start taking care of your skin right away, the effects of menopause can be delayed *and* minimized.'

The women sat up in their seats with eager expressions on their faces. Finally, Dr Rosy felt the connect that was missing in the listless, pessimistic responses she had got earlier.

'How?'

'Before I begin, I want you to remember that the expression you have used the maximum in your life will be the one that will freeze on your face once the wrinkles set in permanently. Those of you who have laughed loud and often will have laughter lines running between your nose and mouth and a crinkling of crow feet at the outer corners of your eyes, which will contribute largely to a pleasing countenance. Those with a grumpy disposition will have deep, vertical frown lines furrowing you forehead etc. etc. So you better start looking your best now, before the look becomes permanent.'

'You have given us something to ponder,' said Leela.

'You know what I think? A face full of wrinkles is a study in history: a lady's life story mapped on her face. Each line has been painstakingly etched by a life experience, giving her face depth and character, while the flawless skin of a young girl is a blank canvas on which life has yet to leave its imprint.'

'That's a lovely way of putting it,' said Sheetal.

'At eighty, my mother-in-law had a beautiful bone structure covered by skin that looked like crumpled parchment. I would be fascinated by the way the creases that crisscrossed her face would increase with fatigue and smoothen out to a certain degree after a good night's rest. But enough anecdotes for now. Let's take up the conditions we are likely to encounter at this age and discuss the ways to minimize them as we go along.'

'Yes.'

'At the outset, I would like to tell you that I have taken the help of my dermatologist friend and most of the inputs I am about to impart are from him. He explained that young, healthy skin has collagen that imparts firmness, smoothness and elasticity. Oestrogen is responsible for this, though the thin film of oil (sebum) that covers it to prevent drying is due to the presence of androgens (male hormones). As I have mentioned in an earlier talk, small amounts of male hormones are present in females and are also responsible for their libido. A decrease in the levels of the above hormones lead to thinning of the skin and loss of firmness and elasticity. A reduction in the blood supply to the skin leads to decreased oxygenation and nutrition. Absence of sebum causes increased water loss and dryness, for the skin is unable to retain moisture. This makes the skin thin, lax, dry, itchy and prone to bruises. Decrease in oestrogen also causes loss of hair in the armpit and pubic area, while the relatively higher levels of androgens (as compared to oestrogens) lead to frontal alopecia (loss of hair from the front of the scalp), unwanted hair on the upper lip and chin and even pimples in some women! The thin, dry skin, without collagen support, causes **wrinkles**; pouches appear under the eyes and large pores become evident.

'However, menopause is not the only culprit and one must consult a doctor, for diseases such as hypothyroidism, fungal infections and vitamin deficiencies also cause skin problems, which can be alleviated upon treatment of the ailment.

'Next to menopause, exposure to the sun is the biggest culprit. A combination of hormonal changes and sun exposure leads to pigmentation on their face, called melasma, chiefly on the cheeks, upper lip and forehead. Age spots develop chiefly on the arms but can be seen in every other exposed body part. Most of our preventive measures are directed towards minimizing exposure to the sun.

'Got it, girls?'

'Yes, ma'am,' they chorused like a bunch of schoolgirls.

'Good,' said Dr Rosy in the same vein. 'As skin changes start as early as perimenopause, your average age group, as I can see, and are permanent, you can accomplish a lot by taking care of your skin from today onwards. So, for a smoother, prettier skin:

♦ Eat foods rich in omega-3 fatty acids. These are found in food such as walnuts, flaxseeds, salmon and sardines. They maintain the skin's oil barrier, which prevents the drying process. Keep yourself hydrated. Avoid alcohol and nicotine like the plague, or should I say like the coronavirus, if you want to prevent premature ageing of your skin.

♦ Liberal use of sunscreen with an SPF of 15 or 30, with UVA and UVB protection, on all exposed areas of the skin, is a must. A beautician patient once told me that the secret to glowing skin is to use sunscreen even at home. I do not know if this helps but what I do know is that exposure to the sun can cause wrinkles, moles and even skin cancers. Use a sunscreen even if the sky is cloudy, for UV rays can penetrate clouds, fog and even snow! Ideally, you must visit a skin doctor before starting any sort of skincare, however innocuous it may seem. Dermatologists usually recommend sunscreen with a moisturizer in the daytime and creams with retinoids (derivatives of Vitamin A) or ceramides at night. You must think that ortho and derma doctors contradict each other but, all that the former asks of you is to expose your face, neck, arms and forearms to the sun for twenty minutes in the forenoon to get vitamin D.

♦ Do not bathe with very hot water even if you feel like soaking in a steaming hot bath to let the tiredness seep away. Take short baths with warm water. You do not have to scrupulously scrub yourself all over with soap for it removes the essential oils covering your skin. Unless you feel really dirty, use soap on areas like your underarms, feet, and groin because the rest of your body is usually quite clean. Scented, antibacterial or deodorant soaps may irritate the skin, so opt for unscented, mild soaps.

♦ Moisturize, moisturize, moisturize as often as you can—after a bath and each time your skin feels dry and itchy. Expensive lotions may soothe your vanity along with your skin, but their poor cousins, like petroleum jelly (Vaseline) and glycerine, work just as well.

♦ Exercise—besides being good for your heart and bones, exercise increases the blood flow to your skin, increasing the flow of oxygen and nutrients to the skin, thereby improving its texture and tone. Like oestrogen, exercise also increases the collagen content of your skin, making it appear youthful.

♦ Yoga—there are yoga exercises especially for the face, which, if practised for even five minutes a day, can decrease/delay the sagging of skin and wrinkles and help retain your youthful look. The earlier you start, the better the results will be. They are easy to perform and include simple things like blowing out your cheeks, shifting the air from one cheek to the other, pursing your lips, raising your head skywards and pursing your lips, twenty times each. You can look them up on YouTube or learn from a yoga guru.

'So you see, a great deal is in your hands, and the time to begin is now if you want to retain that youthful look by natural means. Got it?' said Dr Rosy.

'Yes,' they chorused happily, excited at the prospect of doing so little to gain so much.

'Now let's take up **hairy issues**, the bane of post-menopausal life. As levels of female hormones fall, the small amount of androgens circulating in our system get the upper hand and try to assert themselves by sprouting hair under the chin and along the jaw line or above the upper lip, besides thinning our scalp hair! The first sign will be a widening of the parting of the hair. In some cases, the hairline begins to recede and with it, your sense of self-worth.

'Iron deficiency, anaemia, can cause hair loss and usually occurs due to deficient intake or decreased absorption as the gastrointestinal tract becomes sluggish with age, resulting in malabsorption. Take iron tablets as prescribed by your doctor in case your haemoglobin levels are low.

Hirsutism

For unwanted hair, one could start with milder forms of treatment like depilatory creams, plucking, shaving or waxing. If your skin has become too thin for waxing and tears easily, a visit to the dermatologist is necessary. They may prescribe minoxidil, laser treatment or both. Laser hair removal can work wonders in expert hands. It is also used to remove warts and extra skin tags that tend to sprout after menopause. Hair transplant may be an option for those with severe hair loss.

Now let's take up age spots. If you have been an outdoor person all your life, you will notice age spots in exposed areas and areas of darker skin on your face, hands, neck, arms or chest. Starting now, apply sunscreen with SPF 30 or higher and with UV protection on exposed areas before going out. Existing age spots will fade, new ones will not develop. More importantly, it will reduce the risk of skin cancer.

Dryness, wrinkles and age spots

Do not start any treatment without a derma consult, for sometimes skin cancer looks like a mere age spot! Other signs of skin cancer are the development of a new mole or an increase in the size of an existing mole. Do not delay treatment for it can spread, making it that much more difficult to treat.

Pimples

Surprisingly, some women develop acne, more so on the lower face, after menopause; the culprit again being androgens that take advantage of the decreased/absent oestrogens to assert themselves. As the skin of older ladies is thin, medicines used for teenagers cannot be used for the older population, for they are harsh on older skin. Consult a dermatologist for gentler prescription cleansers and local medications. You might even need oral antibiotics and low-dose oral contraceptive pills.

'Another thing I want to tell you is that wounds heal more slowly, again due to decreased hormones levels. Except for getting yourself tested for diabetes (which again delays wound healing), all you can do is grin and bear it, for eventually, it *will* heal. In the meantime, keep the area clean to prevent infections.

'Lastly, there is the effect of menopause on the delicate skin of the female genitalia. As this area is rich in oestrogen receptors, it is especially vulnerable to reduction in levels during the peri- and postmenopausal period. The thinning (atrophy) of vaginal skin, including its opening (vestibule), leads to a condition called **vaginal atrophy**. This causes itching, tenderness and, at times, a burning sensation in the local area. Intercourse and urination become painful. Avoid use of soaps and do not rub the genital area hard. Apply lubricants to keep it moist. In case there is infection, local or oral antibiotics or anti-fungal medicines may be needed.

Visit a gynaecologist, who will prescribe an oestrogen cream, which is found to be particularly useful in such cases. It is inserted deep inside the vagina with an applicator at bedtime in the prescribed dose.

Skin Changes After Menopause
- Wrinkled, thin and dry skin
- Age spots
- Thinning of scalp hair and appearance of hair on the chin, upper lip and moles
- Warts and moles
- Pimples
- Poor wound healing; easy bruising
- Skin cancer
- Vaginal atrophy

To summarize management:
- Use fragrance-free soaps and moisturizers to decrease skin irritation.
- Avoid exposure to sun; apply sunscreen lotion over exposed areas 20 minutes before going out.
- Adopt a healthy lifestyle that includes adequate exercise, sleep and a balanced diet but excludes alcohol and nicotine. Do yoga regularly.
- HRT, particularly oestrogen, increases collagen content and thereby the skin thickness and smoothness, but is not recommended for skin conditions alone.
- Visit a dermatologist before starting any form of skincare.

17

LOOKING MENOPAUSE IN THE EYE

Aaj agar bhar aai hain
Boondein baras jayengi
Kal kya pata inke liye
Aankhein taras jaayengi
Jaane kab gum hua kahan khoya
Ek ansuun chhupaake rakha tha
Tujhse naraz nahin zindagi
Hairaan hoon main.

(If my eyes fill up today
The drops will rain down
Who knows, tomorrow
The eyes will pine for them
Where has it been lost
The one teardrop I had kept hidden

I am not angry with you, Life,
I am surprised)

This beautiful song from the movie *Masoom* came to her mind as Dr Rosy stood outside the doctor's office with a prescription for artificial tears in her hand. Artificial tears! She did not even know they existed. That there would come a day when she would have to buy tears from the chemist was unbelievable. *She*, who was a sensitive soul and a poet to boot, who cried at the slightest pretext. As she held in her hand the emotionless tears bottled in little green plastic, she smiled wryly and wondered how matters had come to such a pass in this mechanized world of today.

Recently, her eyes had begun to itch. They burned as if sprinkled with grit that wouldn't go away, no matter how many times she splashed her eyes with water. Her inability to resist the urge to rub them had led to redness and watering. Light hurt her eyes and she wore sunglasses even at home to avoid the glare. Dr Rosy thought she had developed eye flu, so when her son came for a visit with his family, she told him to keep the grandchildren away from her lest they catch the infection, though she longed to crush them in her arms and cover their faces with kisses. As she longed to enjoy her time with her loved one, Dr Rosy visited the ophthalmologist that very day.

When he gave his verdict, Dr Rosy did not know whether she ought to be thankful or dismayed. That it was not an infectious eye condition meant that she could play with my grandchildren; this was good news, very good news indeed! That it was a permanent affliction called 'dry eye' was something she would take time to get used to. He told her that this was something she would have to learn to live with, just as she had learnt to live with my diabetes and hypertension. Failing faculties was a part of the ageing process and the sooner she learnt to adjust to them, the better it would be for her.

'Like diabetes and hypertension, afflictions such as these can only be controlled, not cured,' he continued. Alleviation of symptoms was the best he could offer and she could only be grateful for it. Besides the artificial tears, she was told to make some lifestyle changes, to which she readily agreed.

'Dry eye', the doctor explained, occurred in the ageing population of both genders due to a decrease in tear production, and an increase in tear evaporation or production of tears that are ineffective in filming and moistening the eyeballs. Postmenopausal women are more prone to dry eyes as compared to males in the same age group. Sex hormones like oestrogen affect tear production in some way, but the exact relationship is unknown. However, those on HRT, for other reasons, did not seem to benefit from it. In fact, some studies showed that HRT aggravated eye symptoms instead of reducing them.

Women could decrease the incidence and severity of dry eye by avoiding environmental triggers that could lead to quicker tear evaporation. These included:

- Air conditioning
- Dry winter air
- Wind, smoke, pollen
- Outdoor activities

The eye doctor advised, 'If at all you have to go out, they should wear sunglasses that are covered on the sides, to block the entry of wind and dry air into the eye. Try using a humidifier at home or at the workplace. Decrease time spent in front of the computer or the TV, for one tends to stare unblinkingly at the screen for a long time. This causes dryness of eyes, even in the younger population. In case you have to watch the computer screen for prolonged periods, blink frequently, close your eyes off and on and take breaks. Follow the 20:20:20 rule: while at the computer, look at a distance of 20 feet, for 20 seconds after every 20 minutes. Switch over to glasses from contact lenses as they worsen the situation. Moreover, the shape of the eye changes slightly at this age, making the use of contact lenses uncomfortable A diet rich in omega-3 fatty acids and Vitamin A is good for the eyes. You must tell the doctor what medicines you are on, as drugs used for allergy and depression can cause dryness of eyes.'

'Artificial tears forms a film over the eyes and keep them moist,' continued the eye doctor. 'Use them four times a day. Before bedtime, you can use a lubricating gel for long-lasting action. Do not use the gel during the day as the thick coating will blur your vision. These simple measures suffice in most cases. Come for a follow-up visit after a fortnight. If there is no improvement, I will prescribe medicines that decrease the inflammation (redness and swelling) of the eyelids and eyes.'

'In case artificial tears don't work, what then?' she asked anxiously.

'We have drugs that increase tear production, but don't worry—in most cases, artificial tears suffice. In the rare case when all the above fail, we put a tiny insert between the eyelids and the eyeball that slowly releases a lubricating substance throughout the day.'

Prevention Of Dry Eyes
Avoid:

- ◆ Air conditioning
- ◆ Dry winter air, wind, smoke, pollen
- ◆ Outdoor activities
- ◆ Wear sunglasses with side covers that block the entry of wind and dry air
- ◆ Use a humidifier at home and at the workplace
- ◆ Decrease screen time
- ◆ Use glasses instead of contact lenses
- ◆ Eat a diet rich in omega-3 fatty acids and Vitamin A

'Are there complications of dry eyes?' she asked.

'If dry eyes become a chronic condition, it can lead to eye infections, while severe dry eyes can cause pain, corneal ulcer and vision problems.'

'What other eye changes occur with age? Now that I am in your office, could you do a complete eye check-up?'

'I'll be glad to do so,' smiled the doctor. 'However, with the redness and watering, it will be difficult to test your vision today.'

'Never mind, I visited an optometrist recently and got a new pair of glasses.'

'Good. Voluntary preventive health check-up has never caught on with the Indian population, but I try to motivate patients when they come for minor ailments. First and foremost, everyone knows that vision diminishes with age and there is the need for reading glasses. The other conditions we have to look out for at this age are cataracts (*motiabind*) and glaucoma (*kala motia*). The incidence of cataracts (clouding of the lens of the eye) is higher in postmenopausal women than in men of the same age and is usually seen at around sixty years of age. It develops slowly and painlessly, with gradual blurring of vision; there is difficulty in night vision and double vision. The good news is that an operation, during which the damaged natural lens is replaced by a clear artificial lens, restores sight.'

'Do I have cataract?'

'No.'

'Thank God, but I read and write a lot—will that increase my chances of developing cataract?'

'No, but you will become aware of its presence earlier than others because of these activities.'

'One more thing: what is "*kacha motia*"?'

'Perhaps the lay public calls the early stages of cataract kacha motia and think that one should wait for cataract to cloud the entire lens, to "ripen", so to say, before getting it operated. This is a misconception. On the contrary, if the damaged lens is removed in the early stages, the results are much better.'

Cataract
♦ In older population
♦ More in postmenopausal women
♦ Slow and painless clouding of the eye
♦ Gradual blurring of vision
♦ Poor night vision
♦ Double vision
♦ Surgery replaces damaged natural lens with a clear artificial lens
♦ One does not have to wait for kacha motia to 'ripen' before surgery

'Thank you for clearing the cobwebs from my mind. Now could you please tell me what glaucoma is?'

'Glaucoma, or kala motia, as it is called in lay terms, is a condition in which the pressure within the eye increases due to increase in fluid in the eyeball. It occurs equally in both sexes, age being the only contributory factor. It damages the optic nerve, eventually leading to permanent blindness if untreated. As it is painless, people do not realize they have it until the vision loss is severe. The loss of vision begins peripherally, which is not appreciable in the early stages. That is why it is very important to see an eye doctor regularly so that they can check your eye pressure and the status of your optic nerve. Once glaucoma is diagnosed, treatment will be aimed at lowering eye pressure to prevent further damage to the optic nerve and vision loss. This can be done by eyedrops that either increase the outflow of the fluid or decrease the amount of fluid your eye produces. Laser can also be used to increase the outflow. Now let me check the pressure in both your eyeballs.'

Dr Rosy was told to put her chin on a chin-rest and look into a contraption that released a puff of air directed separately towards each eye, which surprised and scared her a bit. However, what mattered was that the pressure in her eye was normal.

Glaucoma
◆   In ageing population
◆   Occurs equally in both sexes
◆   Increases with pressure in the eyeball
◆   Compresses the optic nerve
◆   Leads to permanent, painless blindness

◆	Loss of peripheral vision
◆	Managed by drugs to lower pressure
◆	Laser surgery to increase the outflow of excess fluid

'Please do come for check-ups every six months so that eye diseases are caught in the early, treatable stage,' said the doctor as she got up to leave.

'I will, doc. Sight is precious and I would not like to lose it, especially to conditions that can be prevented.'

'That's the attitude,' said the doctor, giving her a thumbs up.

She vowed to keep my promise, for she did not want to be a burden on anyone. If she took care of my health, she knew that she would have a long, productive life ahead of her, and this is what she produced after wetting her eyes with artificial tears.

Being a woman I have wept
Tears of sorrow, tears of joy
Tears of bitterness, tears of pain
Tears of frustration, fury and fear.
Though, at times my eyes,
Tear up, for no earthly reason
I shed them over
Deaths and disappointments
Failure, loss and broken dreams
Acts of cruelty, act of kindness,
And, for all else that lies in between.
Tears dampen and film my eyes
Or hang, like dewdrops on my lids
They trickle down drop by drop

To merge into scalding rivulets
Or, well from bottomless wells
To gush in tormented torrents
I know that,
With age comes acceptance
That smothers teary responses.
And the twin globes of my eyes
Don't glisten, as brightly, as before.
But the sand that grits behind my lids
And hurts my eyes as if they were
Being pierced with red hot pincers
Give me, not a moment's peace.
Eagerly I delve into the well of
Tears, deep within, and beg it to,
Yield a stream, a trickle, a tiny drop
To quench the embers, burning my orbs
But long since dried, it has nothing to give.
And in desperation I turn
To another merciful soul for help.
But, never did I imagine, that one day
I would stand stunned outside the
Doctor's office, holding in my hand
A prescription for artificial tears!
And from bottled tears, sans emotion,
I seek respite for my tortured eyes.

18

A MOUTHFUL OF TROUBLES

As a novice in dentistry, Dr Ruby (Dr Rosy's daughter and a dentist by profession) had concentrated on excelling in scaling and polishing of teeth, tooth extraction and root canal, for they are the bread and butter of every dentist. Little did she realize that there was more to the mouth than these few simple procedures, more so in the older population, chiefly females, after menopause. What initiated this interest was the mother of a friend, Seema. The old lady, Meera, had come to live with her daughter for a few days. To impress her mother, Seema prepared ice cream, into which she threw a handful of coarsely ground nuts, and impress her she did—in the wrong way. Instead of the cool, smooth sweetness her mother expected to taste, she encountered the unexpected hardness of an almond that bit into a brittle tooth! Instead of appreciating her daughter's culinary effort, her mother angrily exclaimed, 'Who on earth puts almonds in ice cream?' Though hurt, the poor girl said nothing.

A couple of days later, Seema ended up doing the wrong thing once again. She sat with her mom, watching a movie on Netflix in a darkened room with a bowl of deliciously hot, buttered popcorn between them. Seema so wanted it to be a cinema hall experience. They were both enjoying the movie and the popcorn till 'kadak' went another tooth, for her mother had inadvertently bitten into an un-popped corn! She held the broken bit of yet another chipped tooth in her hand and looked accusingly at her daughter, as if the younger woman was bent on reducing her to a toothless old hag!

On the verge of tears, Seema brought her mother to Dr Ruby. On examining her oral cavity, she told Meera that the fault lay with *her* teeth and not with her daughter's cooking! Though teeth are the strongest structure in the human body, stronger than bone, many changes occur for the worse with age, particularly after menopause. However, a lot depended upon the care that was taken of the teeth in the preceding years. Her teeth had become fragile and vulnerable to fractures due to age, menopausal withdrawal of hormones and lack of adequate dental care. Some of her teeth were loose while others had caries that could not withstand the slightest pressure. She would have to get all her teeth removed and once her gums had healed, get artificial ones implanted with the help of an orthodontist.

Dr Ruby said, 'Research, published in Community Dentistry and Oral Epidemiology, has revealed that more than 25 per cent of postmenopausal women are at risk of losing their teeth, chiefly due to bone loss, tooth decay and gum disease. Menopause leads to osteoporosis and in a woman like you, loss of bone in the jaw may initially present merely as a receding gum line. This exposes more of the tooth to decay. Adequate intake of calcium, magnesium and Vitamin D from before the onset of menopause reduces/delays/prevents bone loss, as does avoiding alcohol and smoking.'

'If your teeth feel sore and are getting a little bit loose, visit a dentist at the earliest. A dental check-up every six months, even if there are no dental issues, will prevent many a problem or catch them early, for the risk of dental problems increases with age. At this time, they may feel sore or a bit loose, for which a dental consult is a must. The other changes that can occur in the oral cavity due to menopause and age are:

Dry mouth

A fall in the levels of oestrogen tends to tends to dry up the skin and all the mucus membranes in the body, including the mouth, the nose, the eyes and the vagina. As regards the mouth, women notice that they have difficulty chewing or swallowing food, which may take longer than it took earlier. Talking also dries the mouth and one may have to take a few sips of water before uttering the next sentence. Saliva cleanses the teeth and rinses the oral cavity, thereby removing bacteria. Those with a dry mouth have a decreased flow of saliva flow, increasing the risk of cavities. A dry mouth along with bone loss is double bad news, for teeth begin to fall like nine pins.

After confirming with the doctor that your dry mouth is not due to a blocked salivary duct or a condition called Sjogren's syndrome, which is a combination of dry eyes and dry mouth that needs specialized attention, dryness of mouth can be tackled by:

- ♦ Sucking on ice chips or sugar-free candy
- ♦ Drinking water or other caffeine-free drinks
- ♦ Avoiding salty, spicy, sticky and sugary foods
- ♦ Avoiding dry foods that are hard to chew
- ♦ Avoiding alcohol, tobacco and caffeine
- ♦ Sleeping with a humidifier on in your room might help
- ♦ Using dry mouth spray or rinse
- ♦ Using fluoride toothpaste to help reduce the risk of tooth decay, which increases with dryness

Gums and teeth

Many women in the older age group have receding, sensitive gums that bleed easily on brushing. They need to visit a dentist and inform them that they are going through the menopause. Natural toothpaste with neem may stop bacterial growth in the mouth.

Burning mouth syndrome

This is a condition that comes and goes. During flare-ups, the mouth feels as if it's on fire. It could be nutritional deficiencies, for either the diet and/or digestion is poor at this age, while nutritional needs increase. Supplements are required to make up the deficiency and improve symptoms.

Anaemia could be another reason. Most women who have had heavy bleeding in their perimenopausal period tend to be anaemic and once this is taken care of, oral problems too are relieved. As the burning increases during stress, learn stress-relieving methods like deep breathing, yoga and meditation.

Hypothyroidism could be another reason. If you are feeling low and tired without reason, have sleep disturbances or find changes in the skin, hair and nails, get your thyroid hormone levels checked and start medication if required.

Loss of taste

Postmenopausal women may experience loss of taste as the taste receptors on their tongues are not as efficient as before. As a result, they tend to add more salt or sugar in their food. There may be a genuine increase in the need of salt in women who suffer from hot flashes and cold sweats, but one must be cautious if hypertensive.

Geographical tongue

When the repair of the tongue becomes impaired, it results in a patchwork multi-coloured tongue with painful grooves. Spices, citrus foods, caffeine and alcohol can trigger flare-ups. Zinc supplements help, as does Vitamin B. Reduce stress levels and use milder toothpastes and mouth washes.

Fortunately, most dental issues do not happen overnight. How the teeth and gums respond to age depends, in part, on how well they have been cared for over the years. To minimize the risk of tooth loss during and after menopause, maintain proper dental hygiene.

- ◆ Brush with fluoridated toothpaste and a good toothbrush

- ◆ Floss daily
- ◆ Eat a balanced diet
- ◆ Avoid caffeine, sugar, alcohol and smoking
- ◆ Take your vitamins—C, D, B—plus calcium and magnesium
- ◆ Avoid stress
- ◆ Visit your dentist twice a year

'Last but not the least, I would like to mention the ancient Ayurvedic practice of *kavala gandusha* (*kavala*—oral cavity, *gandusha*—gargle) or oil pulling. This involves swishing a tablespoon of oil (preferably organic coconut oil) in the mouth cavity for 20 minutes to pull out oral toxins. It should ideally be done on an empty stomach. Like the skin, the tongue also removes toxins from the body. As the practice of gandusha pulls out all kinds of built-up toxins from the mouth, it helps in the alleviation of all kinds of mouth, voice and teeth disorders. Besides comprehensive oral and dental health care, gandusha tones the skin of the face, making it glowing and wrinkle-free. It also cleanses the ear, nose and throat and helps treat conditions ranging from sinusitis, migraine and asthma to diabetes. While it's best to do it every day, thrice a week can suffice.'

Changes in The Oral Cavity after Menopause
◆ Bone loss in the jaw
◆ Decay and loosening of teeth
◆ Dry mouth
◆ Receding, sensitive, bleeding gums
◆ Loss of taste
◆ Burning mouth
◆ Geographical tongue

Prevention of Dental Problems
◆ Brush with fluoridated toothpaste and a good tooth-brush
◆ Floss daily
◆ Eat a balanced diet
◆ Avoid caffeine, sugar, alcohol and smoking
◆ Take your vitamins—C, D, B—plus calcium and magnesium
◆ Avoid stress
◆ Visit your dentist twice a year

19

SOME LAST QUESTIONS

This was the last talk that Dr Rosy would be giving in the seminar room of Mascot Enterprises, to a group of ladies who had become dear friends by now. In gratitude, the girls had collected money for a beautiful gift for the kind lady who had unstintingly given them her time and a wealth of information. She had increased their knowledge, cleared their doubts and answered their queries with infinite patience. Her beautiful smile, the fragrance of the flower in her hair and her winning manner would say with them for long afterwards. Both the teacher and the taught were sad. Though they would visit her individually for personal problems, as and when required, there would be no more of such fun sessions.

'Myths abound in every phase of a woman's life,' began Dr Rosy. 'If she begins menstruating (attains menarche, as they say in medical parlance) early, it is because she has been eating *garam* (hot) foods like eggs and non-vegetarian stuff. She is considered unclean during the days she bleeds and is not allowed to enter the temple, the kitchen or do any housework, a custom practised in villages even now. I used to think that it would be a relief to have a compulsory five- to seven-day holiday from drudgery, till the enforced corona holiday taught me otherwise. What I do know is that there is a village in Rajasthan where the mothers-in-law are so fed up of managing the house during the week their daughters-in-law menstruate, that once childbearing is over, the *bahus* are made to get rid of their uteri. There is a doctor in a nearby town who blithely obliges and is minting money doing hysterectomies for such an unethical reason!'

'Oh my God! That doctor should be shot!' exclaimed Meena.

'I wouldn't go as far as that,' smiled Dr Rosy. 'As for pregnancy, there is no dearth of myths. Women are asked to look at pictures of beautiful children so that their baby looks as good as the one they watch, as if genes have no role to play. She is made to drink ghee in milk so that the baby slips out easily. I tell them that they are lubricating the wrong hole! A prevailing myth is that a woman is responsible for the sex of the child and female-producing wives are blamed, even discarded, for this 'aberration', though it has been scientifically proven that the male-producing Y chromosome comes from the male and his wife is just a carrier, so to say. Not all myths are false. I still marvel how our ancestors knew that it takes six weeks after delivery for the uterus to return to its pre-pregnancy state, hence the forty-day *japa* period they insisted on for a woman to recoup from childbirth.

'Interesting as they are, today I will restrict myself to myths associated with menopause:

All sort of problems begin with menopause.

Partly true. Menopause does make a woman prone to heart disease, fractures and senile dementia, but so does age. Men too suffer from similar ailments, though the decrease in hormone levels does add up for women. One can minimize these and even delay them indefinitely by maintaining a healthy lifestyle and a positive attitude.

Menopause brings many symptoms along with it.

Partly true, for there is a wide spectrum of symptoms associated with menopause. However, some women have such a smooth transition from the reproductive to the menopausal phase, with not a single symptom, that makes them wonder what all the fuss was about. Others could suffer anything ranging from hot flashes and cold sweats to genitor-urinary symptoms and weak bones prone to fractures, but there is no need to be pessimistic about it, for they can be managed with medical assistance.

The end of menstruation signals the end of sexual life.

'False,' chorused her bright 'students', making Dr Rosy laugh.

'Yes. We have seen that some women become hornier and hairier after menopause, for testosterone (a small amount of male hormones in the blood responsible for libido) gets the upper hand after the levels of female hormones decrease, thereby increasing sex drive. The inclination for sex also increases because the messiness of periods, the need for contraception and the fear of pregnancy are over, the nest is empty and her partner retired, with all the time in the world at their disposal to indulge in such activities, which makes them enjoy it all the more! There are others who are willing but cannot enjoy sex because of the dryness which causes soreness and pain. Once they start using water-based lubricants or oestrogen-based creams locally, they are as good as new. However, a lot depends on the woman's health, the health of her partner and her relationship with him, besides any sexual issues that have been carried forward. These have nothing to do with menopause.

'A busy life with chronic fatigue, low moods and sleep disturbances take a toll on the sex life of a person of either sex at any age, more so at this age, contributing to a decrease in the desire for sex. Tackling the root cause, for example, by a good night's rest or a short holiday with your partner, can work wonders in replenishing sexual vigour.

You do not need contraception after you stop your periods.

False. Why? Because you do not know that you have attained menopause till a year after the last period. Many women have erratic, delayed cycles in later years and do ovulate occasionally, which can lead to unwanted pregnancies. It is always a good idea to use contraceptives till two years after the last period. Those who have had an intrauterine contraceptive device inserted should not be in a hurry to get rid of it. Others can use barrier methods like condoms, especially with a new or with multiple partners, for sexually transmitted diseases, including HIV, are on the rise in people over fifty. As for contraceptive pills, they are not for postmenopausal women.

You put on weight after menopause.

True to a certain extent: the older you get, the more difficult it is to maintain optimal weight, especially around menopause. Due to hormonal changes, you tend to gain more weight around your abdomen than around your hips and thighs. A lot depends upon your lifestyle and genetic factors. If there is a family tendency to gain weight in middle age, you are likely to do the same. Also, with age, one tends to lose muscle mass due to slowing down of metabolism, while fat increases. If you continue to eat as before but do not increase your physical activity, you will gain weight. You can reverse it by inculcating healthful eating habits and leading an active lifestyle. Lack of sleep may be a contributory factor, for people who sleep less tend to snack more.

'Besides making you look ungainly, increased fat around your middle predisposes you to diabetes, heart and lung problems and certain cancers like that of the breast, colon and endometrial cavity.

'Though postmenopausal weight gain is not shed easily, the formula remains the same—eat less and work out more. Physical activity should include aerobic exercise, like walking for 150 minutes a week, and strength training at least twice a week. The latter increases muscle mass, which helps your body burn more calories. Also, decrease your calorie intake by about 200 once you cross fifty years of age, but do not decrease the nutritional value of your food. Replace processed food and sugars, beverages with empty calories, red meat and dairy fats with a diet rich in fruits, vegetables, legumes, nuts, soy and whole grains. Limit the intake of alcohol. These changes have to be permanently incorporated into your lifestyle. Any slackness on your part will undo the good you have so painstakingly achieved and you will have to start all over again.

Sleep problems have nothing to do with menopause.

False. They do—big time. As many as 60 per cent of postmenopausal women have difficulty in initiating or maintaining sleep. Hot flashes could be one reason; others could be mood disorders or insomnia. To improve the quality of sleep, include some sort of exercise in your daily regimen, and meditate. Avoid caffeine, which can take up to eight hours to be completely eliminated from the body. Try to sleep and wake up at the same time every day. Avoid watching late-night TV shows. Read or listen to light music before going to bed. A warm bath and a warm glass of milk may help. Keep your bedroom cool and comfortable, and wear loose cotton clothes to bed.

Hormone replacement therapy is dangerous.

Partly true. Temporary use of low-dose hormone replacements is safe for the majority of women, but it has to be taken under strict medical supervision. They are particularly useful in treating hot flashes and genitor urinary symptoms like vaginal dryness.

On the other hand, there are women who think all females should be put on HRT after menopause to maintain their youth and prevent its deleterious effect. This is a false notion and could be positively dangerous in women who have a personal or family history of breast or endometrial cancers. It is also contraindicated in women with a tendency for intravascular clotting.

If your periods have begun early in life, they will end early too.

False. In fact, it is the other way around in many cases. They may finish late, though most women will attain menopause between forty-five and fifty-five years of age. Those who have early menopause for whatever reason should visit a gynaecologist as she may need HRT till the actual age of menopause is reached to prevent the side effects of hormonal withdrawal manifesting at an early age.

Menopausal symptoms are only physical.

False. You can get symptoms which are both physical and emotional. You could have mood swings, irritability and become generally disgruntled with life for no reason. You will have to put in extra effort to overcome these by going out and meeting friends, doing regular exercise and eating a balanced, nutritious diet. If you are unable to do it on your own, there is no shame in seeking medical help.

'These are all the myths I could think of,' said Dr Rosy after she finished. 'If there are any you have in mind, feel free to ask me.'

Their hearts were too full to think of such matters and no one wanted to know anything more. It was time to bid farewell to their beloved doctor and they were going to do it in style. After a sumptuous lunch, one by one, each and every one of them hugged her warmly and gave her a potted plant. Looking at the veritable garden by her side, Rosy thanked them from the bottom of her heart, but that was not all. As representative of the entire group, Mona, who had introduced Dr Rosy to her colleagues in the first place, handed her a slim velvet box. It contained a delicate gold bracelet, which the good doctor promptly wore on her wrist.

'I will treasure it for the rest of my life,' she said with tears in her eyes.

20

AND THEY LIVED HAPPILY EVER AFTER

As Meera had guests at home and Shiela would be late from work, they would not be able to join Mona for their evening walk. Both had assured her that they would join her later for their customary gossip session. After all, it was good to share their day with each other and venting was one way to clear the mind of negative thoughts

Mona sat on a bench by the play area of the park watching Myra, her five-year-old daughter play. She was the apple of her eye, the joy of her life. According to Mona, never did a more beautiful, intelligent, loving and lovable child exist on the face of the earth, as all mothers thought of their offspring. She watched Myra happily slide down the slide, swing on the swings and felt blessed. Her mind was replaying happy memories. She had conceived miraculously, spontaneously at around forty years of age when all treatments for infertility had failed, and they had given up hope. And she did not even know! She thought that she had missed her periods due to impending menopause and was happily surprised to learn that she was pregnant. Then followed a tension filled nine months on account of her being an 'elderly primi' (a woman who conceives for the first time at a later age). Such a pregnancy was fraught with complications but as she was fit and healthy and had no co-morbidities like high blood pressure or diabetes, Dr Rosy told tell her not to get unduly stressed.

She remembered the day Myra was born as if it was yesterday. As Dr Rosy had predicted, Mona literally sailed through her pregnancy but what surprised the good doctor was that even as she was planning a caesarean section to decrease the risks, Mona reached the hospital in an advanced labour stage and delivered a baby girl normally within two hours! It was one of the easiest deliveries Dr Rosy had conducted.

'You could have delivered on the way.' She admonished Mona, 'Why didn't you come earlier?'

'I had mild discomfort in my stomach at night. When I confided in Mohit, he said it could be due to the *rajma chawal* we had for dinner, because he too was feeling uncomfortable. It did not occur to me that I was in labour because the due date was a good three weeks away. I had heard horror stories about the intensity of labour pains and these "cramps" were quite tolerable. Moreover, Mohit had them too!' Dr Rosy had burst out laughing.

She could never forget the look of ecstasy on the face of her husband-turned-brand-new-father and love for the two most important people in her life welled from her eyes. Though Mohit loved children, *she* had postponed childbearing for the sake of her career till it was too late but he had never blamed her. She was so very glad that finally she had been able to give him the child he had longed for.

Even as she was thinking such gratifying thoughts, she saw her husband approach the doctor shyly. Overwhelmed with emotion, he asked, 'Can I give you a hug?'

'Of course.' said Dr Rosy and was instantaneously engulfed in a warm embrace.

Mona's parents had come to help during her postpartum period. They insisted that Dr Rosy to give *jaman ghutii* to the child. It was a custom in which the person they wanted the child to be like, puts a drop of honey on child's tongue. This practice was discouraged in hospital but Dr Rosy did not have the heart to refuse. After all, they were bestowing on her a great honour. The first picture Mohit took of the child was with her obstetrician. It adorns the first page of the child's album and is titled 'Rosy with the rose she gifted us.'

When her two friends had joined her on the park bench, Mona said, 'You know what happened at Dr Rosy's clinic today?'

'What?'

'I had taken Myra along and as usual Dr Rosy indulged her. She let her revolve on the revolving stool, listened patiently to her incessant chatter and asked conversationally, "What do you want to become when you grow up?" Myra stopped fiddling with whatever it was on the doctor's desk, stood erect, put her hands on her sides like a soldier and said seriously, "DOCTOR ROSY." The doctor was touched and giving Myra tight hug she said, "Such are the moments doctors live for."'

'So sweet,' said Meera.

After years of turbulence, Meera's life was peaceful. The troubles with her in-law were finally over and she was in a calmer frame of mind. Not that her troubles were of the usual kind—mother-in-law/daughter-in-law wars with the son/husband as the bone of contention. Mataji had been a sweet natured woman who tried her best not to trouble anyone, but troubles had plagued her towards the last few years of her life. First, she had fractured both her wrists, then had to be operated for prolapse and was always apologetic about her dependence on Meera. On her part, Meera had been sincere, kind and caring; and the old lady had blessed her from the bottom of her heart. The last couple of years had been tough as the old woman slipped into dementia and finally passed away. Meera had mourned her as she would have mourned her own mother. Later, her undemonstrative husband had expressed his gratitude by taking her on a trip to Europe. It had always been her life's dream. She could not stop talking about the wonders of London, Paris, Rome, Venice; and her friends did not have the heart to tell her that they had heard her stories so many times before. After all, they were all in that age group when people repeat themselves, and, though this may exasperate their children, the least friends could do was to accommodate those sailing in the same boat.

Age had touched Mona but fleetingly. This could be because with such a young child her joys and worries were of a mother while the other two were grandmothers. Moreover, she was the youngest of the lot. As for Shiela, her left knee had started giving her trouble. The orthopaedic doctor had asked her to do certain exercises, take calcium, Vitamin D tablets and pain killers. He also told her categorically to lose weight added, 'You can't expect a truck to move on the wheels of a Maruti!'

Eventually, perhaps ten years down the line, she would need total knee replacement surgery but she was not unduly worried. She would cross that bridge when she came to it. Who knows, the weight loss could further delay the surgery or she may not need it at all. What mattered was, that the condition had a cure.

Presently, she was in a happy space. The 'dementia scare' had frightened her out of her wits and she was mighty grateful to the Almighty that it had just been 'brain fog'. Thankfully, with the warmth of her friends and the counsel of her doctor, it had almost cleared. She was back to cracking her silly jokes.

'A professor was asked to give a talk on sex. The audience sat on the edge of their seats expecting an interesting discourse on intercourse. On reaching the podium, all the professor said was "Ladies and gentlemen, it gives me great pleasure." and walked back to his seat.'

The friends laughed uproariously, Shiela, the loudest of them all. Her school staff would die of shock seeing their stern ma'am, at the centre of such rollicking laughter. The three were indeed happy. Drunk with the sheer joy of being healthy, carefree and in congenial company, all that they wanted was to remain in such a state of intoxication for the rest of their lives.

ACKNOWLEDGEMENTS

First and foremost, I owe immense gratitude to those patients who came to me during this difficult period of their lives. If I gave them succour, they gave me a wealth of information and an insight into their psyche. Besides their physical symptoms, they discussed with me their fear and phobias, their insecurities and imperfections which, I have put to good use in this book. I thank my colleagues for adding their anecdotes to mine to enrich my writing experience.

I cannot thank Vaishali Mathur enough, for converting what could have been a didactic boring read into a lively one for, she prompted me to write it in the form of a readable, relatable story. Into this format, I wove the stories of three women between their forties and fifties, who could be you, me or anyone else in this age group.

I am grateful to Shreya Mukherjee for painstakingly going over the manuscript with a fine-toothed comb to bring it to its present polished state.

Last but not the least, though I have dedicated the book to her, I thank Sheetal Luthra from the bottom of my heart for helping me fulfil a lifelong dream.

                                        Dr Amrinder Bajaj